AF379076

LIGAMENT AND TENDON RELAXATION
(Skeletal Disability)

TREATED BY PROLOTHERAPY
(Fibro-Osseous Proliferation)

Third Edition

LIGAMENT AND TENDON RELAXATION
(Skeletal Disability)

TREATED BY PROLOTHERAPY
(Fibro-Osseous Proliferation)

By

GEORGE STUART HACKETT, M.D., F.A.C.S.
Consulting Surgeon, Mercy Hospital
Canton, Ohio

With Special Reference to
Occipito-Cervical and Low Back Disability—Trigger Point
Pain, Referred Pain, Headache and Sciatica

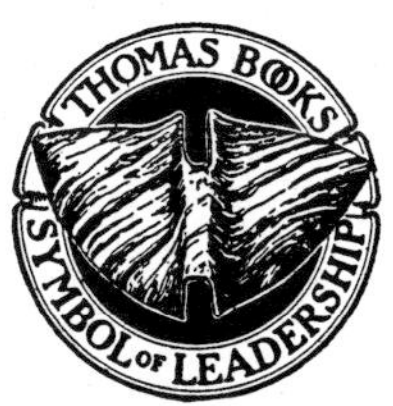

CHARLES C THOMAS · PUBLISHER
Springfield · Illinois · U.S.A.

CHARLES C THOMAS • PUBLISHER

BANNERSTONE HOUSE

301-327 East Lawrence Avenue, Springfield, Illinois, U.S.A.

Published simultaneously in the British Commonwealth of Nations by
BLACKWELL SCIENTIFIC PUBLICATIONS, LTD., OXFORD, ENGLAND

Published simultaneously in Canada by
THE RYERSON PRESS, TORONTO

Printed in the United States of America

PREFACE TO THIRD EDITION

The importance of the work presented in this book lies in the fact that for the first time in history the most frequent cause of chronic painful skeletal disability has been definitely established. A method of confirming the diagnosis and a successful treatment have been developed.

Within the attachment of weakened ligaments and tendons to bone, the sensory nerves become overstimulated by abnormal tension to become not only the origin of specific local pain, but also definite areas of referred pain throughout the body to as far as the head, fingers and toes from specific relaxed ligaments and tendons.

Prolotherapy. A treatment to permanently strengthen the "weld" of disabled ligaments and tendons to bone by stimulating the production of new bone and fibrous tissue cells has been developed.

Adoption of improved diagnosis and treatment of skeletal disability by orthopedic and neurological surgeons will reduce spinal fusion operations to 5 per cent of the peak attained in the postwar devastating decade, just as goiter and mastoid operations were similarly curtailed by the adoption of improved scientific methods. Public resistance has already reduced the operations to approximately 50 per cent because of the high degree of failures which is recognized by both the medical profession and the public. Improved diagnosis will also obviate the exploratory laminectomy operations in search for suspected ruptured disc. Strengthening of the posterior spinal ligaments will prevent many discs from rupturing. Adoption of the treatment outlined in this book will bring permanent relief to millions of sufferers who cannot attain it in any other way.

The previous editions have been completely revised with the inclusion of additional scientific developments to enable the reader to become more competent in the diagnosis and treatment of skeletal disability.

An important addition are ten dermatomes of referred pain and "sciatica" from disabled ligaments that normally maintain stability of the lumbosacral and sacroiliac articulations, and from disabled tendons of lumbar muscles. They are of such practical importance in diagnosis that they will do more to clear up the confusion of low back disability than anything previously presented. They should be included in all future works on low back disability.

Illustrations and descriptions of trigger points and referred pain areas from *somatic tendon relaxation* throughout the skeleton are of especial importance and complement *ligament relaxation* in clearing up the confusion in diagnosis.

A revised illustration of ligaments and their trigger points of pain includes the improved positions for inserting and directing the needles for strengthening the ligaments by PROLOTHERAPY. The technic of treatment is described in detail.

Effective proliferants of new bone and fibrous tissue cells are described in detail as to their preparation, strength, combinations, number and frequency of both office and hospital treatments, together with the aftercare of the patient.

Ligament and tendon disability resulting from operations is fully discussed, including treatment and case reports.

An index has also been provided for convenience.

I am gratified by the widespread adoption of Prolotherapy for skeletal disability by competent physicians in this and other countries, which has made the treatment more available to humanity, and its demonstration to other physicians.

I appreciate the contribution of medical sections and magazines, and the press and radio in bringing this work to the attention of physicians and the awaiting public.

The appreciation and loyalty of patients, visiting physicians, and assistants continues to be an inspiration.

G. S. H.

PREFACE TO SECOND EDITION

As this book goes into its second edition, significant advances in skeletal disability have been included in Part III.

1. Tendon Relaxation as a common cause of disability at the attachment of muscle to bone, particularly in the back, is presented for the first time.

2. A dermatome of referred pain areas into the groin, abdomen, genitalia, buttock and extremities from relaxed ligaments of the lumbar and pelvic articulations directs attention to specific ligaments of the lumbar and pelvic articulations, which are the cause of more chronic low back disability than any other entity.

3. Improved technic which simplifies the treatment of ligament relaxation in joint instability of the lumbar spine and pelvis.

4. A proliferating solution suitable for ligament and tendon stabilization in office treatment.

5. Observations on disabilities resulting from laminectomy, arthrodesis, and cordotomy operations in relation to the original disability of ligament relaxation in joint instability.

G. S. H.

PREFACE TO FIRST EDITION

This presentation has the objective of assembling for the first time the fragments of knowledge that have previously been recorded concerning the disability of articular ligaments and correlating that knowledge with the accomplishments which I have been able to make in the past 16 years while investigating ligament disability from the standpoint of embryology, anatomy, pathology, etiology, symptoms, diagnosis, confirmation of diagnosis, trigger points of pain, referred pain areas, and treatment by a method of strengthening weakened ligaments to re-establish joint stabilization and permanently eliminate pain and joint disability.

It has been my observation that after the early anatomists had dissected, described, named and defined the function of ligaments, they were then taken for granted, and little has been done since to ascertain anything concerning any disability to which they succumb.

The acute disabilities of strain, sprain and torn ligaments have been understood and treated if diagnosed, but there has never been investigation that would lead to an understanding of what, if anything, pathological continued relative to the ligament when recovery was not complete in a short period of time.

This was probably due to the deep inaccessable location of the ligaments, particularly those of the spine and pelvis, for physical examination and the impossibility of detecting them on roentgenograms.

Considerable knowledge has been acquired concerning muscle, bone, intervertebral disc, spinal cord and fluid, and the nerves emanating from the cord. Consequently, any disabilities of the back were attributed to one of the known entities, and much confusion has persisted in diagnosis which in turn resulted in much unsatisfactory treatment.

Further confusion has resulted because, in this highly specialized era, there is a natural tendency for each specialist to fit the symptoms to something in his specialty with which he has some knowledge, or refer them to the neurological or orthopedic specialists. The former know little about and have less interest in the skeleton, while the latter are in the same category relative to the neurological aspects of the low back.

It was, therefore, advisable that ligaments be investigated and presented in a way "that he who walks might see and observe that which is true."

Truth will prevail, and I believe that the main facts in this presentation will endure "as long as man walks on two feet."

To my knowledge this is the first monograph written on ligaments. The fact that ligaments get a portion of a line to show that the author is cognizant of their existance is indicative of the importance with which they are held in disability.

During a period of over 20 years while engaged in a tremendous traumatic practice, I was also regularly called upon for special examinations by approximately 70 accident insurance companies to report accurate diagnoses and prognoses. I became aware of the indefinite and variable conclusions of our best diagnosticians in dealing with low back disability.

Finally, in 1939, I arrived at the conclusion that relaxation of the articular ligaments was responsible for a considerable number of low back disabilities.

I decided to attempt strengthening the ligaments by the injection of a proliferating solution within the fibrous bands to stimulate the production of fibrous tissue.

The treatment proved to be satisfactory almost from the beginning, and it was cautiously extended until now articular ligaments of the entire spine and pelvis and some other joints are treated with great satisfaction both to the patient and to me.

My interest was stimulated to survey all the literature available on the subject of ligament disability. From the meager amount available, I have quoted the important reports on nerve supply to the ligaments and the few reports on tenderness and referred pain areas.

The knowledge acquired from observations while making over 3000 injections within the posterior ligaments of the lumbar spine and pelvis has enabled me to chart trigger points of pain and referred pain areas from individual ligaments which are of inestimable value in diagnosis, verification of the diagnosis, and treatment of ligament relaxation.

In my experience, relaxation of the posterior articular ligaments of the lumbar spine and pelvis are the cause of more low back disability than any other entity. It is also the cause of more referred pain into the lower extremities than any other disability.

A report is made of the animal experiments which have revealed the production of bone and fibrous tissue at the fibro-osseous junction of ligaments from the stimulation of a proliferating solution, when injected within the fibrous bands of tendons. This accounts for the satisfactory clinical results which have been accomplished in joint stabilization by strengthening the relaxed ligaments.

Ligament relaxation is the only condition (disability or disease) in which the diagnosis can both be confirmed before treatment and verified at each treatment.

In this presentation an effort has been made to present it in such a way that any physician may be able to carry out the procedure and at the same time preserve in one article the progress that has been made so that many in the future will have a basis for improving and expanding the diagnosis and treatment of ligament disability.

I desire to express my appreciation to a score or more genuine individuals who recognized the importance of this investigation and made a cheerful contribution that was always an inspiration.

Dr. Donald G. Henderson's preparation of the histological specimens and microphotography are of significant importance.

I am particularly grateful to Margaret Ann Lewis, R.N., my associate as nurse, secretary, statistician and assistant in experimentation on animals, proliferants and anaesthetics. Her cheerful devotion to our objective has been a notable contribution to its success.

G. S. H.

CONTENTS

ILLUSTRATIONS

LIGAMENT AND TENDON RELAXATION
(Skeletal Disability)

TREATED BY PROLOTHERAPY
(Fibro-Osseous Proliferation)

LIGAMENT AND TENDON RELAXATION

"A joint is only as strong as its weakest ligament"—Author

Ligaments supporting the skeletal articulations have been developed over millions of years to provide stabilization of the joints at all positions and limit the extent of motion in all directions.

The early anatomists dissected the ligaments and named them. Since that time, little has been done about them. Their function was taken for granted, and they were inaccessible for obvious determination of continued disability because they could not be observed or palpated and were not revealed on roentgenograms.

For several years I have interviewed medical students and recent graduates from medical schools throughout the country and abroad, and I have been unable to find any medical college in which the deep ligaments of the skeletal articulations are dissected or taught.

Recently I was not greatly surprised to discover, while in conversation with an internationally known surgeon whose name is attached to a type of spinal fusion, that he did not know of the existence of the ilio-lumbar ligament which is important in preventing abnormal movement of the 5th lumbar vertebra on the sacrum and which is usually relaxed in lumbosacral disability. It has a definite trigger point of pain and frequently referred pain areas which are most significant in diagnosis.

In the literature there is an occasional mention of ligaments as being included in the tissues of an articulation, but rarely is there any mention of ligament disability.

At a recent meeting in an internationally known clinic a symposium on "backache" was held in which specialists from the various departments discussed 2000 cases. The cases were divided among 29 different diagnoses, but the word ligament was not mentioned either in the discussion or in the list of diagnoses.

However, a considerable number of the 19 per cent of indeterminate cases were attributed to non-rheumatoid *sacroiliac disease.*

Ligaments are bands of various forms serving to connect together the articular extremities of bones and composed mainly of bundles of white fibrous tissue placed parallel with, or closely interlaced with, one another.

The ligament is pliant and flexible so as to allow the most perfect freedom of movement, but strong, tough and inextensile so as not to yield under the most severely applied force; it is consequently well adapted to serve as the connecting medium between bones.

By the interlacing, crisscrossing and different direction of the bands, the ligaments make it possible for the articulation to withstand strain from any direction. However, the ligaments are frequently placed under acute, continuous or intermittent strain which they are unable to withstand, and their function is permanently impaired by relaxation of the fibrous bands. The bands pass in various directions to support the articulation against stress from any direction while the movement of the joint extends through flexion, extension, or rotation.

Some of the ligaments are connected with the bone as they pass along its surface which enables them to have a firm attachment, while the other end may of necessity be connected with the bone at right angles which makes the junction weaker and more susceptible to separation of the fibrous tissue from the bone. It will be referred to hereafter as the fibro-osseous junction.

In the embryo the mesoderm becomes differentiated into bone, periosteum, cartilage, ligaments, tendons and muscle to serve the individual in the performance of their special functions. However, between the differentiated tissues, there is always maintained a connection by means of white, inelastic fibrous tissue, so that the fibrous tissue of the ligaments and tendons has a continuity through the periosteum with the fibrous matrix of the bone.

As the calcium of the bone encroaches on the amount of fibrous tissue at the fibro-osseous junction of the ligament, there results a weakening of the tensile strength of the ligament as well as a loss of pliability so that the ligament is weaker and more susceptible to injury at that point.

When the fibrous tissue is weakened at the fibro-osseous junction as a result of strain, sprain, tearing or degeneration, the stability of the joint is impaired resulting in a painful disability of ligament relaxation (incompetent).

Ligament relaxation is a condition in which the strength of the ligament fibers has become impaired so that a stretching of the fibrous strands occurs when the ligament is submitted to normal or less then normal tension.

Ligament relaxation was discussed by Meisenbach in 1911 when he reviewed 84 cases of sacroiliac *relaxation*. He stated that, when the tone of the pelvic ligaments is normal, the sacroiliac joints are capable of withstanding much strain, but when they *relax* from any cause, the joints easily yield to strain.

Mengert in 1943 revealed that sacroiliac relaxation was known in antiquity, that it is more common in women, but tends to become more severe in the male. He further observed that it is the function of ligaments to limit the extremes of motion. When muscle assumes the guarding of a *strained* ligament, it becomes tense and fatigued. He also pointed out that the diagnosis of an acute sacroiliac strain is simple during acute episodes but difficult in *mild chronic relaxations,* and it may be advantageous to wait for an exacerbation before attempting a final diagnosis.

Magnuson in 1944 attributed low back pain *more* to strain of the ligaments than any other cause and that there was no place in the body where a differential diagnosis is so necessary as the low back mechanical strains of the lumbosacral area. He stressed that the strains occur not on the intervertebral disc in the low lumbar region but on the ligaments and joints posterior to the spinal canal. The articulations glide and are controlled by the ligaments, and the pains recur after operation when no disc is found.

Ober must have undergone a change of opinion after 1935 when he attributed pain in the cervico-dorsal junction, the dorsal area, lumbosacral, and sacroiliac regions including muscle spasm and sciatica to the pull of the iliotibial band and fascia lata. In 1953 while discussing "lame backs," he said, "Exaggeration of these physiological curves produces mal-alignment resulting in strain of the supporting ligament."

Tendons have likewise been developed as the attachment of muscle at both ends to bone or ligament to act as a cable for the muscular action to be firmly exerted on bone in performance of the special activity for each muscle.

It took about 16 years while dealing with relaxation of ligaments for me to realize that tendons also develop relaxation at their attachment to bone in precisely the same manner. I admit I really felt abashed that it had taken me so long, but I have enjoyed exploring the situation, and I will discuss it as we go along.

In regard to local pain and referred pain, the aim is to establish the source of the somatic pain in the sensory receptors of ligaments and tendons and more particularly in their fibro-osseous attachment to bone, also the definite areas to which the pain is referred from specific ligaments and tendons, and the sciatica resulting from ligament relaxation.

Etiology

Permanent relaxation of ligaments result from strains, sprains and tearing of the fibers as described by Shands. It may occur as the result of a single specific trauma incidental to the strain of an unaccustomed task (Case #1), as when ones foot slips when lifting, or when an unusual great strain is put on a ligament for which it had not previously been developed (Case #2).

It frequently occurs in automobile accidents either alone as a *shearing injury* as I reported in 1954, or in conjunction with fractures, dislocations or other severe injuries.

A *shearing injury* to a joint is one in which the two bones are forced in different directions with sufficient force to stretch or tear the ligaments that normally support the articulation. The shearing action is similar to that which occurs when one blade of a pair of shears is forced in the opposite direction from the other blade.

The shearing accident frequently occurs to the ligaments of the sacroiliac joint in automobile accidents when the automobile is struck either in the front or in the rear, and the victim may be either the driver of the car (Case #3) or a passenger (Case #4) particularly if riding in the front seat.

The mechanism of the injury consists in the forward propulsion of the body including the sacrum while the rigid leg "brakes" against either the foot brake or the floor of the car, forcing the ilium backward; this results in a transverse shearing injury between the ilium and the sacrum. The fibers of the posterior sacroiliac and the interosseous sacroiliac ligaments are sprained or torn.

The shearing action in the sacroiliac joint also takes place when the force is directed in a vertical plane as when one falls in a sitting position on one or both ischial tuberosities, and the force is directed upward through the ilium as the sacrum, with the weight of the torso, is propelled downward (Case #5). The injury to the ligaments may clear up in a few weeks, or it may result in a permanent relaxation of the ligaments.

The shearing injury is occurring with greater frequency owing to the increase of automobiles, speed, stop signs and traffic lights.

When ligament relaxation occurs in a confining injury, it does not give distress until activity has been resumed some weeks or months later and is most likely to be unrecognized because the discomfort is attributed to other factors (Cases #6 and #7). As special examiner for approximately 70 accident insurance companies, I find more than 50 per cent of ligament relaxation cases to be unrecognized following accidents. Some of the cases have had exploratory operations for possible ruptured disc, or had spinal fusion, or both. Often the attending surgeon testifies in court as to the permanancy of the disability when the case could probably be cured in a few weeks by a few treatments of fibro-osseous proliferation.

Ligament relaxation of the low back may be the result of an occupation that requires a lifting, twisting strain in a stooped position, such as that of a housewife (Case #8), farmer (Case #9), industrial worker (Case #10) or an athlete (Case #11).

Often one strain is superimposed upon a pre-existing relaxation which had caused only a slight intermittent disability (Case #12). This may result in a more severe and more constant relaxing disability of the ligaments.

Relaxation of the ligaments supporting the 5th lumbar vertebra frequently occur alone, but in my experience they more often are accompanied by relaxation of the upper portion of the posterior sacroiliac ligaments (Case #10).

Ligament relaxation is occurring more frequently in this mechanized age because our ligaments are not developed to withstand the occasional severe strain to which they are subjected (Case #13). In our modern civilization with mechanized equipment and transportation, the development of the ligaments of our youth is not keeping pace with their skeletal growth, because the child no longer assumes increased family responsibilities of work that would enable them to grow strong. With our mechanical equipment there is not the work to be done. Instead of daily working to obtain spending money, he is given an allowance which he spends at the corner drugstore where he requires only enough spinal stability to prevent his slipping from a stool as he anchors himself with his elbows on the soda fountain counter.

There is no better example of the "passing scene" than the roster of names on "The Irish of Notre Dame" football team. The original fathers of "The Irish" built our railroads, and the sons worked as they grew and developed and later made the team.

When the Irish turned to politics, "The Irish" names on the team were replaced by Italians whose fathers had taken over the maintenance of the railroads. As the Italians took up cement contracting, medicine, law, night clubs, etc., "The Irish of Notre Dame" continues, but the names in the line-up have become a diversity of hard working sons of hard workers. And so it will be.

For several years I have been interested in observing the women of many countries who carry burdens on their heads. Their physicians have informed me that these women never have any trouble with their necks or backs. I have examined them in the doctor's office as they balanced 80 pounds on their heads and moved about with a grace and relaxation which commands admiration. It is because they begin at the age of five years and gradually increase the load as they grow strong.

Ligament relaxation also occurs in the degenerative joint diseases of aging (Case #14) when more strain is placed on the posterior ligament as narrowing of the vertebral bodies and discs occurs.

Newman pointed out in 1952 that weakness of the supra- and interspinus ligaments preceded disc prolapse and that the most common cause of chronic backache is strain on a segment of the spine after the normal checking function of ligaments has been impaired by injury. He further states that it is rational to regard disc prolapse as secondary to ligamentous damage which exists often for years before the prolapse of the disc takes place. In his experience at disc operations the common findings are a torn or inefficient supraspinus ligament and an unstable vertebra.

O'Connell in 1951 attributed low back pain to stretching torn ligaments and advised that "surgery should be reserved for cases in which other measures fail."

Functional relaxation of the pelvic ligaments occurs during pregnancy. Francis in 1951 stated that "During pregnancy the corpus luteum elaborates a hormone called relaxin—permitting the sacroiliac joints and the pubic symphysis to become wider and allowing a greater range of movement—to account for much of the low backache in the late months of pregnancy" (Case #15). Sometimes after parturition the ligaments do not regain their previous tension, and the relaxation persists resulting in chronic low back pain and susceptibility to strains. I have observed many such cases attributed directly to pregnancy, before being cured by fibro-osseous proliferation.

Sometimes a previous ligament relaxation becomes worse during pregnancy or conversely.

Injuries to ligaments have sometimes occurred during shock treatment. There are many cases on record where compression fractures of the vertebrae have occurred. I have treated cases in which a compression fracture of the body of a dorsal vertebra occurred, was recognized and recovery of the fracture took place. However, there remained a painful tender relaxation of the supra- and interspinus ligaments adjoining the spine of the fractured vertebra. They were successfully treated by fibro-osseous proliferation and recovery was complete (Case #16).

Fractures of various bones near the articulations accompanied by torn ligaments result from severe violence. In cases of severe violence just short of fracture, there is frequent tearing of the soft tissues including the ligaments that result in permanent relaxation.

I always look for and frequently find undiagnosed ligament relaxation in cases whose activities have been restricted following severe fractures and where the unrecognized ligament disability is the only one that remains. There are thousands of such cases today. Many have evaded operations which are unsuccessful in such cases.

Ligament and tendon relaxation of the low back as a result of operations may be divided into two classes. (1) Those cases, particularly gynecological, that may have had no pre-operative back disability and were submitted to articular ligament strain during operations while they were anesthetized. It occurs in the Trendelenburg and jack-knife positions particularly in cases with large buttocks. The center of the table should always be lowered for the Trendelenburg position to make a depression for the buttocks, so that the back of the knees against the table will not produce hyperextension of the lumbar spine and cause an abnormal prolonged strain of the lumbar articular ligaments.

In the jack-knife position, the lumbar ligament fibers may be torn by hyperflexion of the lumbar spine when the buttocks are drawn too far over the end of the table while the legs are suspended.

(2) The other class of post-operative joint instability from ligament relaxation are those cases that had ligament relaxation disability for which an operation was performed on the lumbar spine.

They had laminectomies performed in search for a suspected ruptured or "slipped" disc, arthrodesis in an attempt to stabilize a suspected painful joint, and cordotomy in an attempt to cut off from cerebral consciousness both the painful impulses from the original relaxed ligaments and the additional impulses which result from the operations that had been done in the hope of alleviating the original ligament disability.

Unfortunately the spreading, pulling, tearing and excising of ligaments, muscles and tendons that is done to provide a better exposure in disc and fusion operations sometimes leaves the patient not only with the original relaxed painful ligaments but adds more relaxed ligaments and tendons as an additional source of painful disability.

Ligaments at both ends of the incision are frequently torn from the spinous processes of the lumbar vertabrae and sacrum.

The tendon attachments of the sacrospinalis muscle to the transverse processes of the lumbar vertebrae are frequently torn.

I have confirmed the diagnosis of this disability on one side of the spine where there had been no pain previous to the operation (Cases #17 and 18).

The so-called double-jointed patient with hypermobile joints is more prone to ligament relaxation of one or many joints and less likely to have hypertrophic arthritis. The reverse is true of the tight-jointed individual. This is borne out by roentgenograms. The patient with a painful back, negative x-rays, and whose thumb can be adducted well toward the radius when the wrist is flexed, and accompanying fingers that can be hyperextended, will probably have articular ligament relaxation as a cause of the backache. Their elbows and knees can also be hyperextended, and their feet can be flat without necessarily being painful.

I have had hypermobile-joint patients with as many as 14 joints of the spine and pelvis affected with ligament relaxation.

One case had been in three automobile accidents in one of which the car had turned over. There were no fractures (Case #23). Another had submitted to overstrain at unaccustomed work for several months while markedly obese.

Pathology

Joint ligaments are made up of many strands of fibrous tissue which may run parallel or crisscross at various angles to provide stabilization in all positions.

The stretching or tearing of the fibers which result in relaxation takes place principally at the attachment of the ligament to the bone which will be referred to as the fibro-osseous junction.

It is at the fibro-osseous junction that the weakest point of the skeleton is located, and it is weaker where the ligament joins the bone abruptly at a right angle. When separation of the fibers from bone takes place in acute cases of sprain or tearing, there follows an oozing of lymph or blood at the site of injury which heals by the production of fibrin and inflammatory round cell infiltration which develops into fibrous tissue cells and results in permanent strong fibrous tissue attached to bone. There is also a production of bone cells at the fibro-osseous junction in the repair process, as is evidenced by the increased prominence of bone at the site of ligament attachment which can be observed following recurrent sprains or tears of a ligament at the same site as in finger joints and the arches of the feet although no fracture has occurred.

In cases where the healing process is interfered with due to subsequent separation by activity or by deficient repair capacity by the individual, there results a weakness of the attachment which is designated as ligament relaxation. In such cases the healing process can usually be stimulated by the infiltration of a proliferant solution within the ligament that stimulates the production of the normal healing process of round cell infiltration developing into firm permanent fibrous tissue and bone (Fig. 19).

Leriche in 1930, following studies which revealed the rich supply of sensory nerve endings in articular ligaments, advocated the infiltration of the ligaments with local anesthetics for relief of pain in functional articular disturbances after sprains and fractures. Gardner in 1953 reported the abundant supply of sensory nerves in the tissues surrounding joints particularly in the ligaments, and the most effective stimulus to these nerves is in twisting the joints. When joints were opened under local anesthetics, the capsule and ligaments were highly sensitive whereas synovial tissue was relatively insensitive. "With continuous pain, a maintained reflex muscle spasm results." "The inhibition of antagonistic muscles may be so profound as to result in atrophy."

"Joint pain—if mild may be felt in only the region of the joint but if intense may spread and be felt in the entire limb."

Anderson and Laughlin in 1953 concluded that "In the large majority of cases the cause of backache is a pathologic condition in the spinal joints. In other words, backache is simply joint ache." "The anatomy, physiology and pathology of the joints of the back are the same as in the other joints of the body,—and both lend themselves to similar diagnostic approaches and therapeutic measure." Their conclusions are right but would be more pointed to say that *"back pain is ligament pain"* because, as Leriche pointed out, the pain that is elicited on strain is in the nerve supply of the ligaments.

Pain is perceived when normal tension on a ligament stretches the relaxed ligament fibers, resulting in abnormal tension and stimulation of the sensory nerves because the nerve fibers do not stretch. Most joint pain is ligament pain. This will be proven later by injecting a local anesthetic solution within the ligament and abolishing the pain while confirming the diagnosis and later in each treatment.

In acute cases of sprains and torn ligaments, healing takes place by proliferation of bone and fibrous tissue at the fibro-osseous junction. When the tissues do not heal and ligament relaxation results, induced proliferation of bone and fibrous tissue strengthens the fibro-osseous junction, stabilizes the joint and eliminates the disability.

Attention is being directed away from ligaments when we refer to a joint as being sprained or relaxed when in reality it is the ligament that is relaxed.

It is more proper to say that instability of a joint exists as a result of ligament relaxation.

Ligament relaxation of various degrees exist. Some entirely clear up or are not noticeable because of less arduous activities as the individual organizes his life to avoid any action that aggravates his disability.

In more severe cases there may be a lapse of months between attacks of varying severity, and during its presence the pain may vary greatly in severity.

Some articular ligaments of the body and extremities are more often disabled than others due to their exposure to severe trauma which they are unable to withstand.

Those most frequently encountered in the low back are the posterior ligaments of the spine and pelvis including the interspinus, iliolumbar, sacroiliac, sacrospinus, sacrotuberus, sacrococcygeal, hip and also certain ligaments of the large joints of the extremities. Fortunately, most of these ligaments are located so that they can be palpated under certain conditions of muscular relaxation and have definite trigger points of pain to be identified in diagnosis. Also the ligaments are available for needling so that the diagnosis can be verified and the ligaments successfully treated by fibro-osseous proliferation.

Symptoms

The chief symptom of ligament and tendon relaxation is *pain*. The pain is aggravated by activity when tension is placed upon the ligament and tendon and usually subsides when they are not under tension in inactivity.

The pain may be aching in character, or it may be severe and knifelike when movement is attempted.

The general activity of the patient is usually curtailed.

Severe pain or prolonged activity frequently result in muscle splinting and spasm causing the area of pain to be enlarged so that it is impossible to diagnose the disability until after the patient has been made comfortable with rest and analgesics until the muscular pain and spasticity have subsided.

At other times between attacks, the pain has disappeared along with the tenderness so that it is more difficult to locate the trigger point of pain (Fig. 1). It then may be necessary to await another aggravated attack when the patient can assist in designating the area of pain so that the trigger point may be located at the fibro-osseous junction.

There are also frequently associated areas of referred pain (Fig. 9), particularly if the relaxation is severe. The extent of the referred pain varies greatly for different ligaments (Figs. 2-11).

As a result of the dearth of knowledge about ligament and tendon pain and disability, there has existed a great confusion in the diagnosis and treatment of back disability. It has been the custom for each specialist to someway attach the significance of it to his field of endeavor. Consequently, many patients have received various diagnoses for the same condition, much to the disappointment of the patient as he went the rounds of physicians and practitioners of various cults. I have known patients with curable ligament relaxation of the back to consult over thirty physicians.

Low back pain in the lumbar area may persist for an indefinite time, even years, without any referred pain except "across the back" when there is relaxation of the supra- and interspinus ligaments, which occurs frequently. When these ligaments are relaxed, there is permitted an increased pressure on the intervertebral discs and the bodies of the vertebrae because both lie anterior to the fulcrum which is located in the articular processes while the ligaments lie posterior (Fig. 13). This increased pressure on the disc may result in narrowing of the disc or compression of the disc in such a way as to force the nucleus pulposis through the posterior longitudinal ligament giving rise to the increased symptoms of radicular pain, as the "ruptured disc" produces pressure on the segmental nerve. This is the only explanation for such cases as reported by Alpers in which low back pain is experienced in most cases of herniated lumbar discs and in some instances precedes the appearance of leg pain by up to five years.

Also in 1925 Steindler revealed that "of all the structures entering into the formation of the lower back, i.e., the region of the lumbosacral and sacroiliac junctions, the ligamentous structures are, in response to mechanical agencies, the first to suffer pathological changes."

Of 213 cases analyzed by Steindler, 58.5 per cent were sacroiliac, 36.5 per cent were lumbosacral, 5 per cent were combined, and only in the postural group was lumbosacral predominant. I can add that my experience and observation are similar.

Thus the evidence appears to be conclusive that relaxed supra- and interspinus ligaments are an etiological factor in the occurrence of ruptured disc. If this conclusion is correct, then strengthening the supra- and interspinus ligaments should assist in preventing ruptured disc. When iliolumbar ligament relaxation is also present, it should also be stabilized by fibro-osseous proliferation.

When the low lumbar pain is relieved or absent following disc operations, it is because the operator has removed the supra- and interspinus ligaments along with their nerves. To make up for this loss of tissue, the wound is closed in as many as four layers, each containing about 15 interrupted silk sutures which results in a fibrous scarified area between the erector spinae muscles and is usually free from pain (the nerves having been removed). However, there is frequently pain and tenderness at both ends of the incision which was not present before the operation. This is due to ligament relaxation which resulted from the great force put on the ligament attachments by the muscle spreader and position on the table during the operation while getting a better exposure. If this new post-operative pain does not subside after several weeks, it can usually be eliminated by fibro-osseous proliferation of the ligaments as I have done on many occasions.

Sciatic nerve pain accompanied by tenderness, pain on stretching, radiating pain as far as the toes accompanied by parasthesias, diminution of ankle reflex, ½ to 1 inch muscular degeneration of the thigh and leg (from disuse or impaired nerve function) and body list is due to relaxation of the ligaments that support the lower portion of the sacroiliac joint (Figs. 5, 8, 9).

Pain (Trigger Point Pain, Referred Pain, Sciatica)

The conscious perception of pain in ligament and tendon relaxation has its origin in the sensory nerves which lie within the fibrous bands, particularly at the fibro-osseous junction, where the relaxation most frequently occurs and where the nerve supply is abundant.

The normal function of these sensory nerves, according to Brain, is proprioceptive sensibility appreciation of posture on movement of the body itself, which he attributed especially to muscle, tendon and periosteum. It is my contention that these somatic proprioceptive afferent sensory impulses arise chiefly in the ligaments, which crisscross and run in various directions to maintain stability of the articulations in all positions.

The afferent impulses from the ligaments enter the spinal posterior root ganglion. Under normal conditions many of these proprioceptive impulses do not reach consciousness, but are concerned in reflex activities at the spinal level, or influence the cerebellum in its control of movements and posture. There are related afferent and efferent impulses of the muscles and tendons.

When a normal ligament is submitted to excessive traction or strain at its fibro-periosteal junction, the sensory impulse is of such intensity that it reaches consciousness and a release of traction is voluntarily accomplished.

When the fibrous strands of the ligament become relaxed or weakened from any cause, a normal tension on the ligament causes a stretching or elongation of the fibrous strands of the ligament, and this elongation permits an abnormal tension-stimulation of the intraligamentous nerve fibrils which will not stretch. This is the cause of the local or trigger point pain in ligament relaxation.

The causative factor of the sensory stimulus is tension on the free nerve endings or spindles. Lennander observed in 1901, while operating under local anesthesia, that pain and referred pain resulted from traction on nerves in the pedicles of abdominal organs. *Somatic pain* is the conscious perception of a displeasing sensation from intensified sensory stimuli of somatic origin. Patients differ in their description of the unpleasant sensation which they perceive from a certain ligament, and the sensation may vary in the same patient according to its intensity. This is also true of referred pain and "sciatica" associated with ligament relaxation. They may describe the pain as dull, aching, sharp, piercing, burning, boring, drilling, shooting, numb, dead feeling, itching, pricking, squeezing, compression, pressure, tired, heavy, or pulling.

A brief weak stimulation usually results in local pain only, but when the stimulation is prolonged and/or intense, there is often an accompanying referred pain.

It has become necessary to understand the mechanism that is taking place in the origin of somatic pain. We can no longer accept as accurate the clinical observations that are without scientific basis. Much of the literature including our text books must be rewritten.

Trigger Point Pain: Trigger point pain is an area of hypersensitive somatic sensory nerve receptors that respond more readily and with increased intensity to stimuli of pressure and tension. They are circumscribed in a definite area depending upon the number of ligament and tendon fibers that are relaxed. They are extremely important in diagnosis for (1) locating the exact ligament or tendon causing the pain, (2) confirming the diagnosis by needling, and (3) precisely placing the needle for prolotherapy.

Referred Pain: Sir Henry Head first used the term "referred pain" in 1893. It was my good fortune to have served him as house physician in The London Hospital in 1916. His meticulous examinations have remained an inspiration, and my observations on referred pain would hardly have been made without that association.

The early scientific work on referred pain dealt chiefly with its origin in the nerves of abdominal organs and viscera from which it was referred to somatic structure and skin.

Baer in 1917 associated referred pain into the outerside of the thigh from sacroiliac disability. I visited European clinics with him in 1925.

Steindler and Luck in 1938 in referring to low back pain pointed out, "There is little in the literature to answer the question of specific allocation of pain: where and in what tissues does it actually originate." By needling and procaine injection there was identified definite pain in somatic tissue.

Steinbrocker in 1941 revealed that often the advancing needle will strike the deep trigger point and the pain of which the patient complains is duplicated in quality and radiation. He further stated that this relationship is confirmed by the injection of five cubic centimeters of 1 per cent procaine solution at the spot. The pain and even disability is abolished for several hours or longer.

Travell and Travell in 1946 pointed out that pain in sacroiliac disability may be referred throughout the sciatic distribution into the buttock, outer thigh and leg to just above the malleolus, and that "referred pain induced from injection or needling of trigger points persists for several minutes and its distribution can usually be clearly delineated by the subject."

None of these observers apparently realized that the origin of the pain and *referred pain* was in the ligaments and tendons.

I shall not discuss the many theories that have been suggested to explain referred pain, except to say that it may be due to an induced heightened excitability of nerves and cells which receive impulses from the same spinal segment.

When the ligament fibers become relaxed, a normal tension will then produce a bombardment of afferent somatic proprioceptive sensory impulses from the ligament into the spinal posterior root ganglion where some are transmitted to the brain as consciousness of local pain, while other impulses in some way stimulate exteroceptive impulses which also enter consciousness as superficial pain from an area which has its sensory distribution from the same spinal segment and is known as the *referred pain.*

Individuals with ligament relaxation differ greatly in their susceptibility to referred pain. The intensity and extent of the referred pain varies in the same individual from time to time due to the intensity and duration of the stimulation at the fibroperiosteal junction.

Some patients with ligament relaxation in which the pain is severe, extensive or of long duration may not have any referred pain.

Usually patients with a low pain threshold have more severe and extensive referred pain areas. The high pain threshold patient who has rarely ever had a headache is less likely to have much referred pain and may require more treatment than their complaints would indicate.

It is difficult for some patients to realize and admit they have been benefitted by treatment as long as a considerable discomfort remains from a portion of a ligament or some other cause in the same area. Other patients can readily estimate that they are 50 per cent, 70 per cent, or 90 per cent cured.

When I began my investigation and treatment of ligament instability in 1939, I did not realize that either the local or referred pain had its *origin* within the ligament.

From observations while reproducing and temporarily obliterating pain by intraligamentous needling with a local anesthetic solution, and permanently obliterating both local and referred pain and "sciatica" by strengthening relaxed ligaments, I have been able to correlate definite areas of *referred pain* with specific ligaments of the lumbar and pelvic articulations, and definite areas of *conducted* sciatic pain which had its origin from pelvic articular ligament relaxation.

Some of my earlier presentations have been slightly modified due to additional observations.

The present dermatomes of referred pain areas (Figs. 2 to 11) from specific ligaments (Fig. 1) have been made from observations while giving approximately 18,000 intraligamentous injections to 1,656 patients over a period of 19 years. I believe they will endure as long as man walks upright.

The referred pain areas from ligament relaxation of the lumbar and pelvic articular ligaments do not conform to the skeletal dermatome which have been observed in our text books.

It has been my observation that the referred pains from low back articular ligament relaxation usually are not present to any important degree in the immediate region of the joints in the extremities. This is particularly true at the knee joint, where pain and tenderness due to sciatica are frequently present and of diagnostic importance as will be pointed out later.

Many investigators of referred pain have worked from the area of reference, through the spinal posterior root ganglion, in endeavoring to establish the point of origin of nerve receptor stimulation in an organ or somatic structure which had its innervation from the same spinal posterior segment.

For the relief of referred pain, much effort has been expended by others in endeavoring to interrupt the pathway of impulse.

Our approach in locating specific areas of referred pain has been direct, by the insertion of the point of a needle *within* the fibrous strands of a specific ligament and the injection of a local anesthetic solution. The irritation of the needle and the pressure-tension of the anesthetic solution immediately reproduced the local pain, as in dentistry, and frequently the referred pain, only to disappear within two minutes as anesthesia took place.

Outlining the area of referred pain has been accomplished by the assistance of the patients in pointing out the extent rather than depending on the point of a pin.

The concepts of the Englishmen, Ross, Head and Mackenzie, on cutaneous hyperalgesia as a result of reference from organ and visceral stimulation were not as simple as they were once believed. I have found a definite connection between pain of *somatic origin* from relaxation of ligaments to have a referred manifestation in organs and viscera, such as pain in head, shoulders, arms and fingers from cervical ligaments, gastric distress from mid-thoracic ligaments, and large bowel distention and constipation from iliolumbar ligament relaxation which cleared up when the ligaments were strengthened by Prolotherapy. Although these are valuable observations in explaining some existing symptoms, they do not have the diagnostic importance of the referred pains into the lower extremities, which are also of somatic origin.

With the dependence on x-rays and other modern methods of diagnosis together with the neglect in knowledge of ligament disability, the source of pain which is essential for accurate diagnosis has been overlooked. Consequently, the modern diagnostician with his limited powers of perception is distinctly at a disadvantage.

Now that the greatest source of somatic pain in the lumbar spine and pelvis has been solved and dermatomes of referred pain into the groin, lower abdomen, genitalia, buttock and extremities have proven to be of inestimable value in the diagnosis of low back disability, it is logical to conclude that further investigation of referred and reflex stimulation of ligament and tendon origin will be found to affect the sympathetic nervous system in arteriospasm, to influence the oxygenation and metabolism of tissue as a reflex neurovascular sympathetic disorder such as occurs in Sudeck's post-traumatic acute bone atrophy. According to Bonica, Sudeck's Atrophy was described in 1877 by Wolff, Kummell in 1895, classically by Sudeck in 1900, and as a trophoneuritis in 1902 by Kienbock with accurate roentgenographic description of bone changes. I have observed it to accompany articular ligament relaxation following acute sprain, and to clear up following fibro-osseous proliferation of the ligament. Now that a cause has been identified, many cases in the future can be prevented and the duration of others shortened.

Sudeck's Atrophy may also account for muscle spasm that takes place while sleeping and disappears when the patient awakes, and either by changing position in bed or on arising, the somatic painful stimulus is eliminated and the discomfort subsides.

It accounts for the pain low in the buttocks that occurs after sitting in a chair or automobile when there is tension on relaxed ligaments that prevent backward rotation of the lower portion of the sacrum. A similar pain across the upper sacral area that is present after sitting and clears up on standing is due to muscle spasm accompanying relaxation of the articular ligaments that prevent the forward rotation of the upper portion of the sacrum. The accompanying reflex muscle spasm prevents the patient straightening up and walking until after a brief period when the spasm subsides.

On account of the neurovascular disorder that is associated with early articular ligament disability such as sprains and tearing of the fibers, there is an interference with the normal process of fibro-osteal repair, and an aggravated stimulation of the sensory stimuli will tend to delay the repair process. Consequently, inactivity of the articulation following injury to the ligaments is advisable.

Since ordinary existence of the individual makes inactivity of the articular ligaments of the low back and extremities more difficult to attain than the upper torso and extremities, it is only natural that so much chronic disability of the low back is found. Recognition of this fact should lead to more enforced restricted activity following acute articular ligament disability than has been the custom.

The injection of a local anesthetic into the ligaments of an ankle for relief of pain following an injury may be advisable when accompanied by immobilization and elevation, but if given to enable an athlete to continue activity, the procedure is to be deplored.

Sciatica: In my experience while diagnosing and treating 1656 patients with chronic low back ligament disability, sciatica has been found to have its origin more often as a result of relaxation of the ligaments that support the lower portion of the sacroiliac joint than from all other causes combined (Figs. 1,C,D,SS,ST; 8). The chief cause is relaxation of the lower outer portion of the posterior sacroiliac ligament that is attached to the margin and outer side of the ilium just above the sciatic foramen, where the sciatic nerve emerges in contact with the piriformis muscles. They are all bound together with a fibrous sheath. Relaxation of the ligament is accompanied by spasm of the piriformis muscle which may become inflammatory and swollen along with its sheath so that it can readily involve the trunk of the sciatic nerve, either by mechanical pressure or tension or by extension of the inflammation into the sheath or the nerve. Or it may be affected by a reflex arteriospasm of the inferior gluteal vessels as described by Leriche.

The point of excitation may be on the first, second and third sacral nerves which lie on and are surrounded by the fibers of the piriformis muscle and its tendon within the pelvis before they join the sciatic nerve.

The piriformis muscle has its origin in tendons attached to the anterior surface of the sacrum between the first, second, third and fourth anterior sacral foramen and grooves leading from the foramen along which the sacral nerves pass. According to Bonica, the piriformis muscle bridges the sacroiliac joint adjoining the posterior sacroiliac ligament anteriorly, at the joint margin, and slightly posteriorly.

According to Grant, the sciatic nerve passes above the piriformis muscle in 0.5 per cent of cases, through it in 12 per cent, and below it in 87.5 per cent.

The anterior sacroiliac ligament is undoubtedly relaxed along with relaxation of the posterior sacroiliac ligament, and this would be an additional source of somatic pain stimulation to affect the piriformis muscle and the sciatic nerve, or the sacral nerves before they join the sciatic nerve.

Some fibers of the sacrospinus and sacrotuberus ligaments are also attached in the same area to contribute their additional nerve stimuli.

According to Lewin, rectal examination revealed that straight leg raising stretches the piriformis muscle long before the sciatic nerve could be stretched. Thus, an inflamed capsular membrane of the combined structures could induce sciatic pain by traction.

Sciatica caused by ligament relaxation is a neuritis, and the pain into the lower extremity is *conducted* as an impulse through the nerve from the point of excitation and is not a referred pain.

Although the trigger point tenderness of the sciatic nerve and areas of distribution of conducted pain are constant when recurring in the same individual, there is frequently some variation in other individuals. This is due to a variation in the location and nature of the origin of pain stimulation.

The orgin may be located at any of the sacral nerves before joining the trunk, or different sections of the trunk may be involved.

Trigger point tenderness at the point of emergence of the sciatic nerve through the sacral foramen is usually more intense when sciatica is present along with tenderness of posterior sacro-iliac ligament relaxation and piriformis muscle spasm.

Sciatic tenderness just lateral to the tuberosity of the ischium is more diagnostic. Tenderness throughout the posterior thigh is usually more vague. Of particular value diagnostically is pain and tenderness on palpation of the sciatic nerve in the popliteal space, because it is significantly present when "sciatica" extends below the knee (Fig. 5).

From the main branch of the sciatic nerve in the center of the popliteal, the conducted pain of "sciatica" may cause a severe gripping pain in the calf of the leg and to a less extent in the Achilles tendon and a compression of the heel which is distinct from the referred pain beneath the heel that has its origin in the sacrospinus and/or sacrotuberus ligaments. Pain may extend across the internal malleolus and as a pressure beneath the arch of the foot medially. From the common peroneal branch in the outer popliteal space, the pain may extend down through the anterior medial edge of the tibia, across the tip of internal malleolus, on the top of the foot, and extend into any or all of the toes. The pain from the two branches may combine to give a severe gripping pain in the calf of the leg.

I cannot emphasize too strongly the *necessity of studying* the dermatomes of referred pain and sciatic pain (Figs. 2-11) from specific ligaments together with the ligaments and their trigger points of pain (Fig. 1), so that they will become a *part of your thinking* while obtaining the history and making the physical examination of patients with low back disability.

Diagnosis

The diagnosis of ligament and tendon relaxation at any skeletal location depends on obtaining a history of the disability, followed by a physical examination, and concluded by a confirmation of the diagnosis.

History: The history should include the age, occupation, sex, dates of confinement, duration of disability, cause of disability if known, whether continuous or recurrent, how long disabling and to what extent, whether any compensation is being received or any claim and litigation is involved. Reports of x-rays. Previous operations, treatment, medication and their effect. Menopausal history, bowel elimination, headaches and nervous condition. What activities are prohibited by pain and which induce the pain and its location. Have patient point with *one* finger to the spot of most pain if possible. Statement of weight and if obese, the weight at age 20, and the most ever weighed.

In the cervical area determine if the pain is central and more to one side, and whether the pain extends upward to the occiput or beyond to either side of the head or out toward the shoulder, arm or hand and fingers, and which side is the more severe.

Concerning back pains, learn especially the exact location, whether only in the center, or only on one side, or alternating for a time on one side, then on the other, and if on both sides which is worse. If there is pain in the sacral area when arising after sitting, have the patient stand up and point to the area of

TRIGGER POINTS OF PAIN AND NEEDLES IN POSITION FOR CONFIRMATION OF THE DIAGNOSIS AND FOR TREATMENT OF LIGAMENT RELAXATION OF THE LUMBOSACRAL AND PELVIC JOINTS.

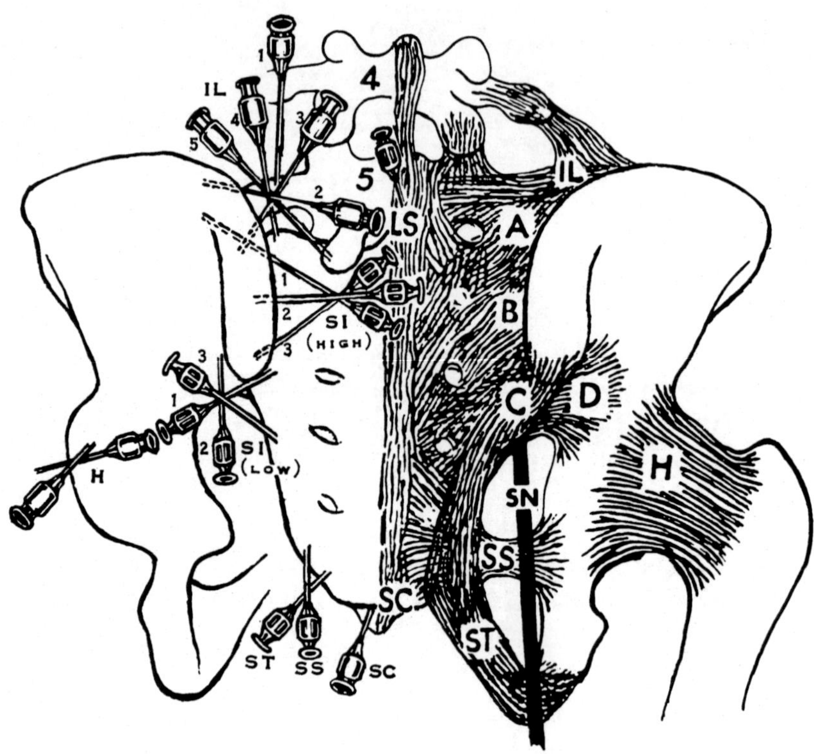

TRIGGER POINTS OF LIGAMENTS

IL	**-**	**Iliolumbar**
LS	**-**	**Lumbosacral - Supra & Interspinus**
A,B,C,D,	**-**	**Posterior Sacroiliac**
SS	**-**	**Sacrospinus**
ST	**-**	**Sacrotuberus**
SC	**-**	**Sacrococcygeal**
H	**-**	**Hip - Articular**
SN	**-**	**Sciatic nerve**

Figure 1.

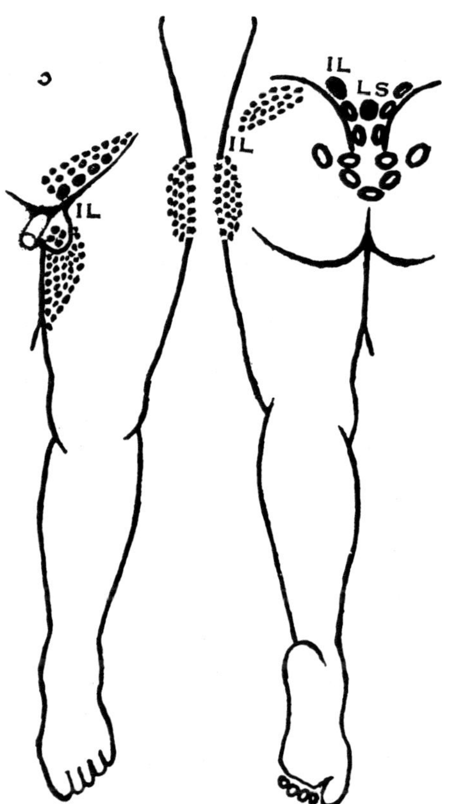

FIGURE 2. ILIOLUMBAR LIGAMENT.
Referred pain areas (IL) are located in the groin, anterior medial upper two-thirds of the thigh, lower abdomen above Poupart's ligament, testicle of the male, vagina in the female, upper buttock beneath the crest of the ilium and upper outer thigh.

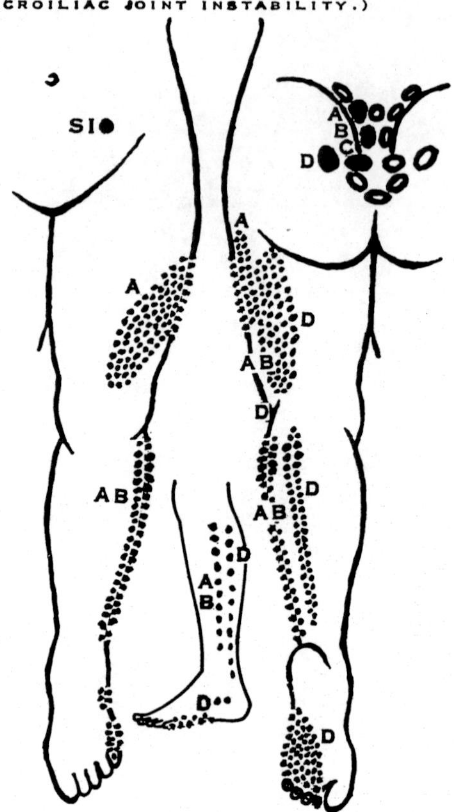

FIGURE 3. POSTERIOR SACROILIAC LIGAMENT.
Referred pain areas from the upper fibers
(Fig. 3-AB) are located on the outer posterior
thigh and extend around anteriorly to the
upper margin of the patella. Below the knee
they extend down the outer side of the leg in
the tibial line to within two inches of the
external malleolus.

From the lower fibers at the inferior margin of the joint on the outside of the ilium
and sacrum (Fig. 3-D) the areas are located
in the posterior thigh, down along the outer
side of the calf of the leg, beneath the external
malleolus, along the outer side of the foot
to the little toe, and sometimes as a numbness
beneath the foot into the four smaller toes.

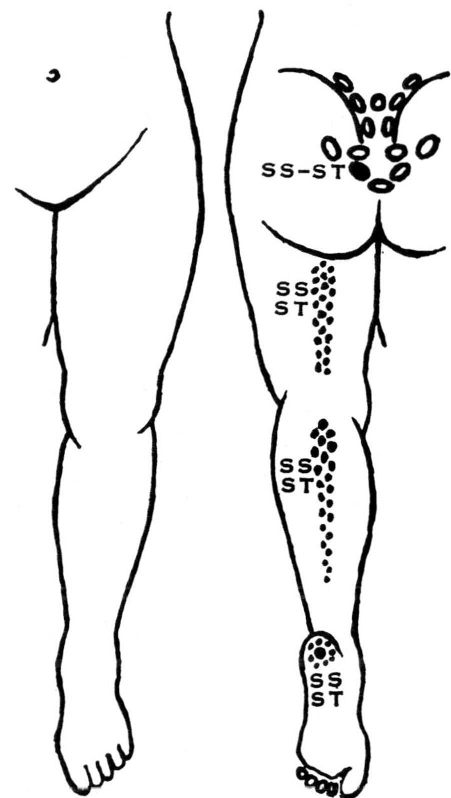

FIGURE 4. SACROSPINUS AND SACROTUBERUS
LIGAMENTS.

Referred pain areas (SS-ST) extend down the
central posterior thigh, down the center of the
calf of the leg, and beneath the heel.

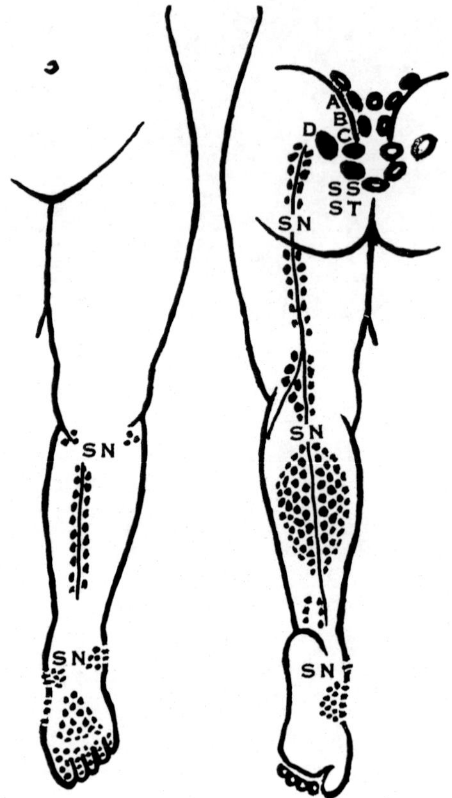

Figure 5. Sciatica

Pain (SN) is conducted (not referred) downward through the buttock and posterior thigh. In the popliteal space there is one pain through the center and another laterally. There may be a pain on either side of the upper end of the tibia which sometimes extends through like a metal pin. In the leg there is a gripping pain in the calf and a vertical pain along the medial edge of the tibia. A pain on either side of the Achilles tendon and on either side gripping the heel.

At the ankle the pain runs across the external malleolus, on the inner side beneath and anterior to the internal malleolus. They may give a feeling of compressing the ankle. Beneath the arch of the foot medially. On top of the foot extending into any or all of the toes, but especially into the great toe.

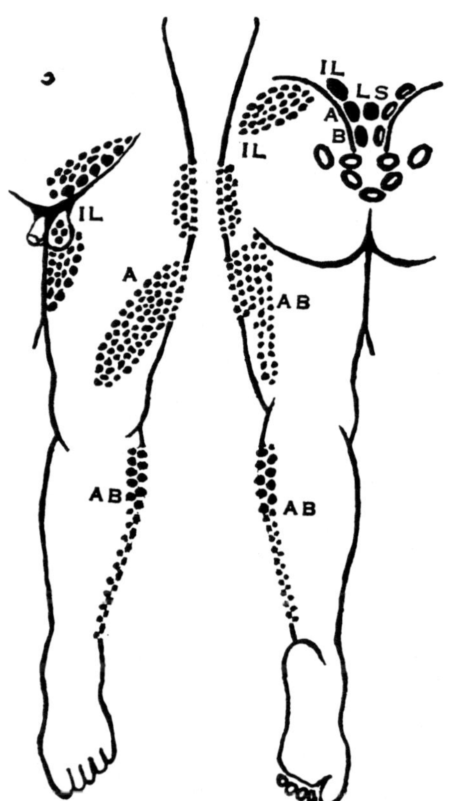

FIGURE 6. ILIOLUMBAR AND POSTERIOR SACROILIAC
(UPPER) LIGAMENTS.

Relaxation of the ligaments of the lumbosacral and
upper portion of the sacroiliac articulations occur together so frequently that their referred pain area from
Figure 2-IL and Figure 3-AB are combined in one dermatome.

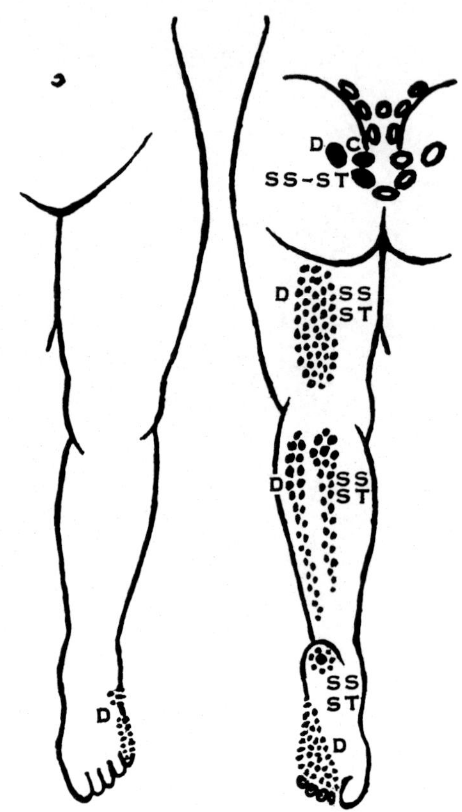

FIGURE 7. POSTERIOR SACROILIAC (LOWER), SAC-
ROSPINUS AND SACROTUBERUS LIGAMENTS.

Relaxation occurs together so frequently that
their referred pain areas from Figure 3-D and
Figure 4-SS-ST are combined in one dermatome.

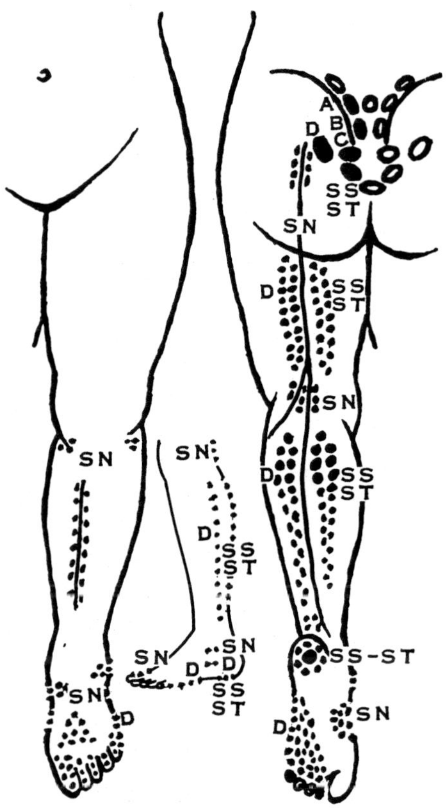

FIGURE 8. POSTERIOR (LOWER) SACROILIAC,
SACROSPINUS AND SACROTUBERUS LIGAMENTS,
AND SCIATICA.

The conducted pain of sciatica (Fig. 5-SN) are illustrated in one dermatome with the referred pain of the sacral ligaments (Fig. 7-D-SS-ST) with which it is always associated.

REFERRED PAIN AND SCIATICA – ILIOLUMBAR, POSTERIOR SACROILIAC, SACROSPINUS AND SACROTUBERUS LIGAMENTS.
(LUMBOSACRAL AND SACROILIAC JOINT INSTABILITY.)

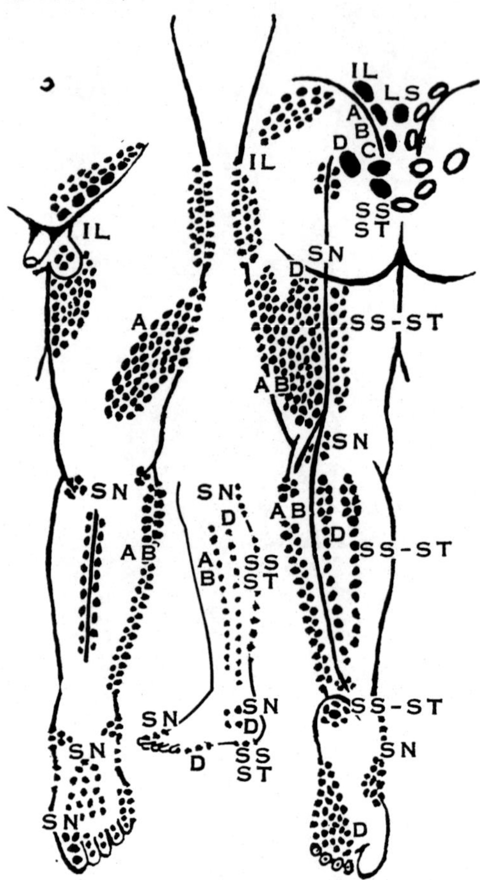

FIGURE 9. REFERRED PAIN OF ILIOLUMBAR, POSTERIOR SACROILIAC, SACROSPINUS AND SACROTUBERUS LIGAMENTS, AND SCIATICA.

Referred pain areas from the iliolumbar (Fig. 2-IL) and sacroiliac (Fig. 3-A,B,C,D), articular supporting ligaments (Fig. 4-SS-ST), along with the conducted pain of sciatica (Fig. 5-SN) are combined in one dermatome.

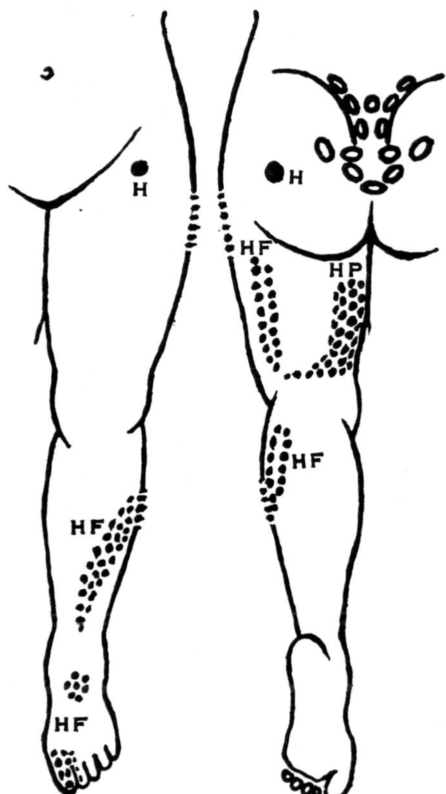

FIGURE 10. HIP ARTICULAR LIGAMENTS.

Referred pain from the pelvic attachment extends down the postero-medial thigh (HP). From the femur attachment there is an area in the postero-lateral thigh (HF), the outer side of the upper calf of the leg which extends around the outer side and down the front of the leg, appears on the top of the foot and into the great toe and half of the second toe.

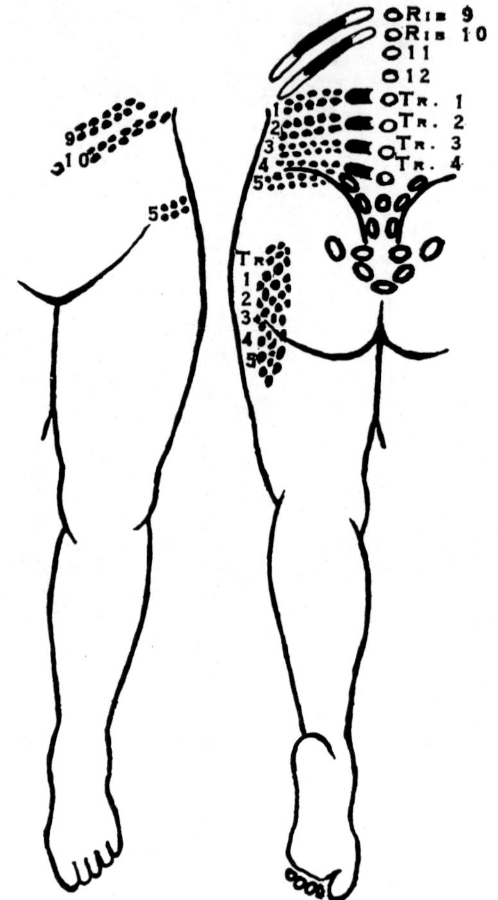

FIGURE 11. ILIOCOSTALIS AND SACROSPINUS TENDONS.

The referred pain areas (1-2-3-4-5) (9-10) and trigger points of pain (Tr. 1-2-3-4-5) (Rib 9-10) from relaxation of tendon attachments of the iliocostalis muscles to the ribs (Rib 9-10), and the tendon attachments of the sacrospinus muscle to the transverse processes (Tr. 1-2-3-4-5) of the lumbar vertebrae are included in one dermatome.

most intense pain. If it is near the top of the sacrum, attention will be directed to the lumbosacral and upper sacroiliac area (Fig. 6). If the pain is in the lower or central area of the sacrum, attention will be directed to the lower sacroiliac joint area and the ligaments which support it (Fig. 7).

Inquire particularly in regard to referred pain from any portion of the spine or pelvis. Concerning low back pain, learn whether the referred pain is felt to extend into the groin, low abdomen, testicle, or vagina. Find out exactly what portion of the thigh, leg, foot and toes the referred pain area involves.

Inquire particularly if the pain is definitely felt in the popliteal space, for this is one of the most important points in determining whether sciatica accompanies the referred pain from the ligaments. The sciatic pain appears in the popliteal space, while referred pain from ligaments is not present in the immediate knee area. In fact, it can be stated that referred pain from ligaments has a tendency to "skip" the larger joints of both the upper and lower extremities.

An experienced examiner, while questioning patients about the referred pain areas particularly in the lower extremities, will form a mental picture of which side and just which particular ligaments or portions of the ligament are most involved in relaxation. The knowledge gained is of great value during the physical examination which follows by directing attention to the seat of disability. The history is so informative that frequently during the interrogation of a patient, I will point out to a visiting physician the particular ligaments which should be involved to account for the pain, and usually the physical examination will verify the conjecture.

Inquire as to which movements induce the pain, and have the patient point to the area. When brushing the teeth, ironing, sweeping, leaning over the washbowl or sink, or putting on the shoes induces a *central* pain in the low back, it is almost a certain indication of relaxation of the ligaments that support the lumbosacral joint. The same movements inducing pain on one or both sides of the low back indicates sacroiliac joint instability.

Of course, conditions other than ligament relaxation will induce these pains, but since articular ligament relaxation causes more low back pain than any other entity and more referred pain into the extremities and sciatica than all other conditions combined, we must consider it in all cases of low back disability, just as appendicitis must be considered in all abdominal disorders.

In patients who have had operations on the lumbar spine, inquiry should reveal whether there exists a lumbar pain extending outward on either or both sides to the outer margin of the back which may or may not have existed prior to the operation. It is indicative of relaxation of the sacrospinalis tendon attachments to the spines laterally and the dorsal surface of the transverse processes of the lumbar vertebrae which frequently has its origin in separation of the attachment by dissection and traction during the operation (Fig. 11).

The patient should always be questioned about bowel elimination, especially if there are a variety of painful areas about the skeleton. A constipated patient (there are many) is almost impossible to cure.

The Physical Examination: Many patients who have often been examined for back disability remove their clothing and lie prone on the examining table. From conversations about previous examinations including post-operative cases, I have come to the conclusion that the physical examination of back cases is a lost art.

Where the ligaments are covered by muscle as in the cervical, lumbar and pelvic portions of the skeleton, it is absolutely necessary to place the patient in a position in which he will be comfortable and have the overlying muscles entirely relaxed. Only then will the examiner be able to make the desired pressure on the ligament that will put tension on the fibers of the ligament with enough intensity to enable the patient to respond that you are pressing on the right place. Never ask the patient if you are producing *the pain* because he will be expecting to perceive the severe pain and you may only be producing a lesser amount. *Always* ask him if *that is the place* or to tell you when you *get to the place* where he has been having trouble, as you go gently from one trigger point to another for comparison. Remember or mark the spot, and come back to it again for confirmation.

Do not poke, punch, dig in, or press hard enough to cause discomfort in a patient without disability, or both you and the patient will become confused.

Examination of the knee and ankle reflexes are important in the examination of low back disability and are influenced by severe ligament relaxation as they are in disc disability.

Muscular degeneration occurs in ligament relaxation as a result of disuse when the painful side of the pelvis is favored for a considerable time by less use of the lower extremity on the affected side and more often when sciatica results from ligament relaxation.

Parathesias of the feet and toes occur in ligament relaxation as in disc disability.

Many leg tests give a variety of painful reactions and lead to confusion. Extension of the flexed leg at the knee while the patient is seated is a good test for pain in the sciatic nerve. In doubtful cases, the test should be made while the patient is reclining. Full rotation of the hip while the patient is lying on his back with the knee flexed (Patrick's sign) is an excellent test for disability of the hip joint and is frequently positive in relaxation of the ilio-femoral (articular) ligament accompanied by trigger point tenderness at the posterior superior area of the articulation.

In the joints which have only a slight superficial covering of soft tissue such as the acromio-clavicular, elbow, wrist and ankle, the trigger points are readily accessible and are located with very little difficulty.

Frequently the patient has such severe ligament pain accompanied by muscular spasticity and pain that the area of tenderness is enlarged, and it is impossible to obtain relaxation of the overlying muscles. In such cases, it is impossible to locate the trigger points, and the patient is treated by rest, analgesics and heat until the acute symptoms have subsided.

At other times the pain and tenderness of one ligament obscures a lesser disability in another ligament which will become troublesome only after the original ligament has become stabilized.

Sometimes between attacks the pain and tenderness are so quiescent that the diagnosis can be made only with great care and skill. In such cases it is well to have the patient return for examination during the next attack.

Have the patient point with *one* finger to the area at which he has his most pain. Palpation in this area will indicate the exact trigger point of pain from ligament or tendon relaxation. Of course, a knowledge of anatomy is necessary to determine its significance. The entire area of relaxation can be outlined by palpation and may be marked with a pen, especially in the spine and ribs areas.

Determining the extent of the area of ligament or tendon relaxation to the occipital bone is simple (Fig. 25). Also the attachment of the deltoid tendon to the acromial process of the scapula and to the outer side of the humerus (Fig. 26), the acromio-clavicular ligaments (Fig. 19), the tendon and ligament attachments of the elbow (Fig. 20), and the ligaments of the wrist (Fig. 21) and ankle (Fig. 23).

Relaxation of the tendon attachment beneath the curved line of the occiput is associated with pain in the eye, temple, headache and dizziness. It has been reproduced by pressure and needling and has cleared up by strengthening the fibro-osseous attachment.

There has also been reproduced by needling a referred pain from the dorsal ligament of the wrist to a point on the shoulder just posterior to the acromial process of the scapula.

Relaxation of the tendon attachments of the supraspinatus and infraspinatus muscles on the dorsal surface of the scapula (Fig. 26) usually cover a larger area and can be readily outlined by palpation.

The tendon attachments of the iliocostalis and other muscle attachments to the ribs are (Fig. 26) easily outlined on the dorsal surface of the ribs when tendon relaxation is present and usually cover an area from 3 to 5 inches long. The back examination can be made while the patient is relaxed standing, seated, and reclining prone.

The cervical and upper dorsal spine examination can usually best be made while the patient is seated astride a chair with his hands or arms resting on the back of the chair (Fig. 12). The examiner stands behind and to the left of the patient. His left hand is placed beneath the chin to obtain complete relaxation of the neck muscles and to make movements of the head that will enable detection of trigger points of both ligaments and tendons.

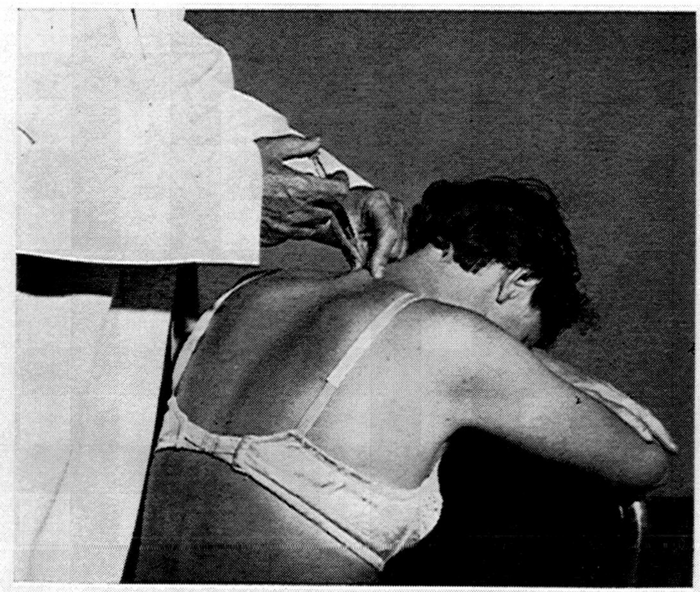

Fig. 12. Patient seated astride chair for occipital, cervical and upper dorsal diagnosis and treatment including "whiplash injuries." Left thumb and index finger astride the supraspinus ligament between spines.

The tenderness of supra- and interspinus ligament relaxation can be elicited either by pressure with the thumb between the spines, or sometimes better by compressing the interspinus spaces between the thumb and index finger (Fig. 13). Deep pressure just lateral to the interspinus spaces will frequently elicit pain when the spinus articular ligaments are relaxed along with the interspinus and the patient has complained of pain just lateral to the spine and often radiating or referred up into the head, out into the shoulder area, arm, forearm and fingers and around the chest to the sternum or abdomen.

The lower dorsal and lumbar spine including the lumbo-sacral and upper sacroiliac ligament disability can best be examined with the patient standing completely relaxed, eyes looking straight forward, hands and fingers hanging free. Brassiere and shorts are usually worn, but no clothing can be supported by the fingers.

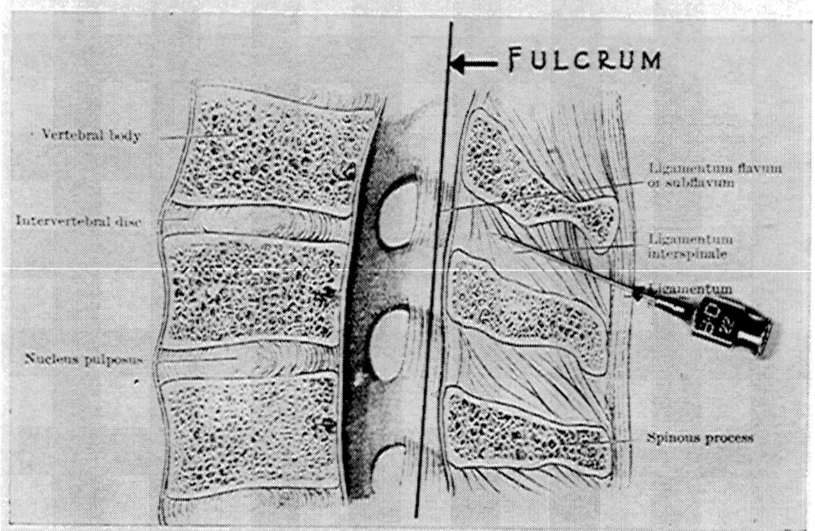

Fig. 13. Vertical section through lumbar vertebrae. Vertical line passes through the two articular fulcrums. One and one-half inch needle in position for confirmation of the diagnosis and for treatment.

The point of the needle has passed through the supraspinus ligament and is in the *diagonal* fibers of the interspinus ligament.

When one vertebra normally glides forward on the articular processes of the adjoining vertebra below, both the interspinus and supraspinus ligaments assume a more diagonal position without stretching, as the spines of the two vertebrae come slightly closer together.

To permit any abnormal forward movement of one vertebra on another such as occurs in spondylolisthesis and compressing an intervertebral disc, the fibers of the interspinus ligament must be torn or stretched, as in chronic relaxation, while the supraspinus ligament may assume a more diagonal position in the moderate cases but must also be disabled together with the spinus articular ligaments and others in the severe cases.

The interspinus ligaments are probably the most important ligament throughout the spine in limiting joint motion while maintaining joint stability.

The interspinus relaxation is frequently accompanied by relaxation of the articular ligaments on one or both sides of the same vertebra.

Ligament and tendon relaxation of the lumbar spine and pelvis are so intimately associated, their ligaments crisscross in some places, and they are so frequently disabled simultaneously with conflicting symptoms that it is best to consider them as components of one area, which I prefer to designate as the *low back.*

To facilitate locating the trigger points of pain over specific relaxed ligaments by palpation and to locate the point at which the needle is to be inserted in confirmation of the diagnosis and in treatment, I have made a sketch of the *landmarks* (Fig. 14) which I use automatically and repetitiously in orientation.

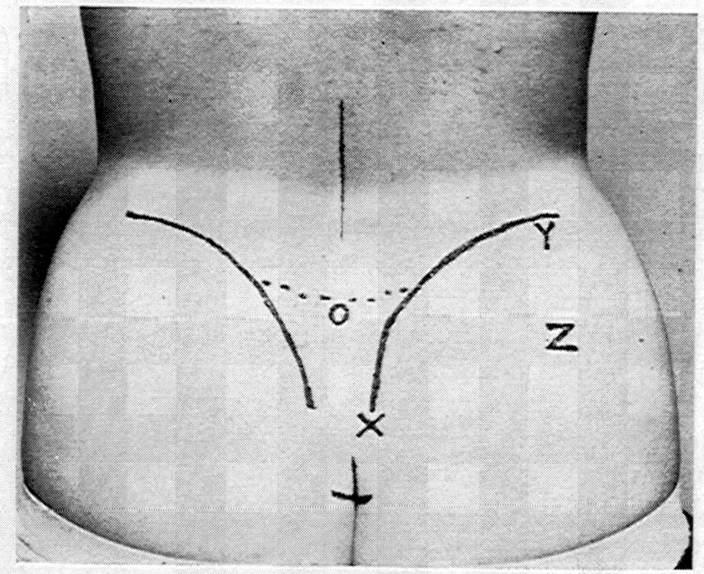

Fig. 14. Bony landmarks for orientation in location of trigger points and needle insertions in the lower lumbar and pelvic ligament.

  O — Lumbosacral depression.
  ------ — Top of sacrum.
  Y — Crest of ilium.
  X — Depression below the posterior spine of the ilium.
  —+— — Bottom of the sacrum.
  Z — Depression at hip joint.
  NOTE: The top of the sacrum is *higher* than the lumbosacral depression.

The curved line beginning at Y is palpated with the index finger to locate the crest of the ilium, while it is followed downward by rolling the thumb over the edge medially to locate the trigger point of the iliolumbar ligament (Fig. 1,IL) just medial to Y. From there on down to X the upper portion of the posterior sacroiliac ligament is located in the same manner by rolling the thumb.

Figure 14,X is the *depression beneath* the posterior superior spine of the ilium. It is a more definite *spot* than the spine which is curved like the top of a mountain. The depression is located by palpation with the thumb.

The midline is located by palpating the lumbar spines above and the sacral spines below with the thumb or index finger and also by observing the crease between the buttocks.

The lumbosacral depression at O is located by pressure with the thumb and is more readily found by gliding the thumb gently upward over the sacrum until it "drops into" the depression between the 5th lumbar and 1st sacral spines.

The bottom of the sacrum is located by palpation with the index finger on the transverse (——) low on the buttock.

These landmarks will be referred to throughout the presentation of diagnosis and treatment of the "low back."

Have the patient indicate with *one* finger the location of the pain while standing *relaxed.*

The diagnosis of relaxation of the supraspinus and interspinus ligaments of the lumbosacral joint (5th lumbar) is one of the easiest to make in the low back.

It is made by pressure with the thumb in the lumbosacral depression, trigger point of pain, Figure 14,O. Avoid strong pressure which will produce pain in most patients. Preferably make gentle increasing pressure while asking the patient if that is "a place" he has been having trouble (avoid using the word pain). Make the thumb pressure at various trigger points (Fig. 1) going slowly and gently from side to side, higher and lower, to compare the suspected trigger points, while asking the patient to inform you when the involved ones are located. The cooperation of the patient is most important, and he should be so informed.

If the muscles become spastic during the examination, have the patient bend slightly forward and straighten up again to the erect relaxed position.

Frequently glance at the patient's head and hands to check on relaxation. It is the *rare* patient who will continue with head erect and arms hanging free without being reminded more than once.

Relaxation of the lumbosacral (5th lumbar) ligaments seldom exists without accompanying relaxation of other ligaments. The most frequent are the following: posterior sacroiliac (upper portion, Fig. 1,A), iliolumbar (Fig. 1,IL), 4th lumbar (supraspinus and interspinus), caspular ligaments of the articular processes, and the sacrospinalis.

Certain body landmarks (Fig. 14) are frequently used to keep orientated while locating the trigger points in diagnosis, and later for inserting the needle in confirmation of the diagnosis and in treatment.

Bimanual pressure is made equally with the left hand against the upper abdomen while with the right thumb, gentle but firm pressure is made at the various trigger points between the spines of the vertebrae, the lumbosacral depression (Fig. 1,LS) for relaxation of the supraspinus and interspinus ligaments, and at the trigger points medial to the curved crest of the ilium (Fig. 1,IL) for relaxation of the iliolumbar ligament attachment to the anterior surface of the ilium just beneath the crest, and for relaxation of the upper portion of the posterior sacroiliac ligament (Fig. 1,A). As pressure is being made with the thumb at the above trigger points, it may help to quickly push backward with the left hand on the lower end of the sternum. As muscle relaxation in the low back results, the thumb more readily reproduces the trigger point pain.

It must be remembered that trigger point tenderness lateral to the lumbosacral depression (Fig. 1,LS) is due to relaxation of the posterior sacroiliac ligament (Fig. 1,A). Its fibers extend upward and outward above the top of the sacrum to be interlaced with the iliolumbar ligament attachment to the ilium, while the spine of the 5th lumbar vertebra extends downward over the top of the sacrum, thus placing the lumbosacral depression and interspinus ligament tenderness below the top of the sacrum. This anatomical relationship has remained confusing because it has never been stressed in medical education. It probably is the greatest cause of mistakes in the diagnosis of low back disability.

This is particularly true because relaxation of the posterior sacroiliac ligaments is the most frequent single cause of low back disability. It occurs in the ratio of 5 to 3 with lumbosacral disability, although some medical centers during the past 25 years have erroneously taught that nothing of significance happens to the sacroiliac articulation.

Occasionally the referred pain areas will be reproduced on pressure over the trigger points in severe cases.

The trigger point pain indicative of relaxation of the lower portion of the sacroiliac ligament (Fig. 1,C,D) and the sacrospinus and sacrotuberus ligaments (Fig. 1,SS,ST), sacrococcygeal ligaments (Fig. 1,SC), and hip articular ligament (Fig. 1,H) and the trigger point pain of sciatic neuritis can more readily be located while the patient is lying comfortable in the prone position with the buttocks completely relaxed.

A trigger point tenderness of the posterior sacroiliac ligament is below and beneath the posterior superior spine of the ilium (Fig. 1,C). The important trigger point (Fig. 1,D) for relaxation of the posterior sacroiliac ligament at the inferior margin of the sacroiliac joint is located by placing the thumb beneath the posterior superior spine of the ilium and moving it slightly outward while making slight pressure upward. The thumb will be felt to pass slightly upward and drop into the groove between the sacrum and ilium where the ligament passes below the joint from its sacral attachment to the ilial attachment, as it forms the margin of the great sciatic foramen medially and above. The trigger point extends over this area of attachment to both bones and is combined with sciatic nerve tenderness and piriformis muscle and tendon tenderness when they are also present.

As the thumb is moved downward along the outer margin of the sacrum, the trigger point tenderness of the relaxed sacrospinus and sacrotuberus ligaments (Fig. 1,SS,ST) are identified.

The ligaments are always relaxed and tender in severe cases of sacroiliac joint instability and especially when accompanied by "sciatica." The trigger point tenderness of the sacrospinus and sacrotuberus is often difficult to produce, but by comparison with pressure on both sides of the sacrum low down toward the coccyx, the patient will usually report a difference.

The trigger point pain of the sacrococcygeal ligament relaxation is located by pressing the thumb over the lower margin of the sacrum (Fig. 1,SC). Pressing the tip of the coccyx forward and backward with the forefinger in the rectum produces pain at the articulation and is the best method of examination because any other abnormality of the coccyx can also be noted.

Pressure over the course of the sciatic nerve in the buttock as it passes downward just lateral to the tuberosity of the ischium is frequently productive of tenderness as compared to the opposite side when sciatica is present. There are two trigger points of the sciatic nerve tenderness in the popliteal space (Fig. 5), and they can best be located with the patient lying on his abdomen with the knees flexed between 45 and 90 degrees and supported with one hand or forearm or by an assistant. The two points are located in the center over the main branch of the sciatic nerve and on the outer side just medial to the tendon of the biceps femoris muscle. The lateral tenderness is over the common peroneal branch of the sciatic nerve.

Pressure just medial and below the top of the greater trochanter of the femur will produce the trigger point pain of relaxation of the articular ligament of the hip (Fig. 1,H).

Diagnosis of tendon relaxation on the dorsal surface of the lumbar transverse processes is made with the patient in the prone position with a pillow under the abdomen. Pressure is made from the outer portion of the lumbar area by the thumb pressing down and medially against the ends of the transverse processes (Fig. 11). Each process can be distinctly differentiated because the process lies transversely outward from the interspinus space immediately below the vertebra to which the process is attached, except the fifth which is very slightly higher and is also shielded by the crest of the ilium. The diagnosis of all of the transverse processes are readily made and verified by inserting a 2 to 2½ inch needle vertically at the point 1-inch lateral to the tip of the left index finger which is placed in the interspinus space.

While locating the trigger points of any of the ligaments and tendons of the skeleton, it is advisable to first press on an area nearby where there is probably no tenderness, so that the patient will be able to compare normal tissue to painful tissue. Then, go from one trigger point to another and back again. A good point to start in examining the sacral ligaments is in the center of the sacrum low down where there is rarely any trigger point pain.

Confirmation of The Diagnosis: Relaxation of ligaments and tendons is the only condition of disability or disease in which the diagnosis can be confirmed before treatment and verified at each treatment.

The technic of verifying the diagnosis consists of selecting a 22 gauge needle, of sufficient length for the particular ligament or tendon, attached to a syringe containing a local anesthetic solution. At the trigger point of pain the point of the needle is inserted within the ligament, and 2 to 5 cubic centimeters of the anesthetic solution is distributed within the ligament throughout its depth. The irritation of the needle alone or together with the pressure of the anesthetic solution will immediately stimulate the production of the pain, and the patient will inform the physician "that is the place." Sometimes the referred pain will also be reproduced.

Two minutes after the needle is withdrawn the patient will be able to move about and go through motions without pain that he was unable to do before. He will realize that the seat of his trouble has been located for the first time. His confidence has been won, and he readily accedes to the treatment advised.

As the physician becomes more experienced, he will be confident of his diagnosis following the history and physical examination. He can then omit the anesthetic solution, and the diagnosis will be confirmed when the needle is inserted for treatment and the pain is reproduced. This method eliminates an extra insertion of the needle which is always appreciated by patients.

As long as any disability remains the pain will be reproduced on inserting the needle. Often the history and physical examination at a later check-up will indicate further treatment of a particular ligament, although the patient believes that area is cured. When the pain is reproduced, the patient will readily agree that the treatment was advisable.

The differential diagnosis between ligament relaxation of the lumbar and pelvic articulations complicated by sciatica and a protruding intervertebral disc with pressure on the radicular nerves is quite simple when one thoroughly understands the referred pain from low back articular ligaments and is competent to reproduce the specific trigger point of ligament pain for each referred pain area by pressure with the thumb and by needling.

The conducted pain of sciatica may be the same whether it originates in the radicular nerve of a spinal segment before joining the sciatic nerve, or on the sciatic nerve as it emerges from the pelvis. Both may have sciatic tenderness and pain on stretching, pain to as far as the toes, loss of ankle or knee reflex, muscular degeneration of the thigh and calf, and body list.

The important point is that when sciatica is caused by relaxation of the ligaments that support the lower portion of the sacrum, there will be trigger point tenderness of the lower portion of the posterior sacroiliac ligament (Fig. 1, D) and of the sacrospinus and sacrotuberus ligament (Fig. 1, SS,ST). Every surgeon who operates on the spine should have a conferee that is competent to diagnose the case for him unless he fully understands ligament disability.

Roentgenograms

Roentgenograms are usually without value in the diagnosis of ligament relaxation, but they are of value in identifying congenital and acquired deformities and bone lesions. However, roentgenograms are only an adjunct to be used in diagnosis just as the thermometer and stethoscope. I have observed that too much importance was attached to apparent abnormalities revealed by x-rays that could not possibly account for the symptoms and signs.

I strongly recommend the procedure which was insisted upon by Stimson* who had practiced orthopedic surgery before the days of roentgenology and which I have followed for 40 years. Always arrive at a tentative diagnosis following a history and physical examination *before* viewing the roentgenograms.

Lowman reveals that joint instability results from ligament deficiency and that by the age of 40, 90 per cent of all persons have degenerative changes in their weight bearing joints.

After comparing roentgenograms of patients without back pains with those with back pains, Bistrom concludes that routine roentgenograms were of little importance in the evaluation of back pain. Splithoff arrived at the same conclusions regarding roentgenograms of the lumbosacral junction.

X-rays to be of diagnostic value must *conform* to the physical examination. Too often the questionable or possible cause of the disability as pointed out by the roentgenologist cannot possibly account for the disability, for its location does not conform to the trigger point areas, and the symptoms obtained in the history also could not possibly conform.

For many years I have observed physicians who are without the ability to diagnose back disability awaiting the decision of the roentgenologist as to the cause and then proceed to carry out an unsuitable course of treatment which is costly in time and money to the patient and to the hospital which is short of beds.

Usually the patient can give a good report on the x-rays that have been taken by the various physicians, specialists, hospitals, and clinics, and most often they are interpreted as negative, minimal arthritis, possible slipped disc, or a vague congenital deformity that had not given any trouble for possibly 35 years.

It has been my observation that exercises strengthen muscles, but further weaken ligaments and tendons when they have become relaxed. Furthermore, the patients cannot carry out the exercises because of the pain which the exercises induce. The illustrations of exercises that are brought to me by patients,

---

*Lewis A. Stimson: Professor of Orthopedic Surgery, Cornell University Medical College, circa early 20th Century.

which they have received from otherwise reputable institutions and specialists, are ludicrous when associated with the disability for which they were prescribed.

Treatment—Prolotherapy

The treatment consists of the injection of a solution *within* the relaxed ligament and tendon which will stimulate the production of new fibrous tissue and bone cells that will strengthen the "weld" of fibrous tissue and bone to stabilize the articulation and permanently eliminate the disability.

To the treatment of proliferating new cells, I have applied the name *prolotherapy* from the word "proli-" (Latin) meaning offspring; "proliferate"—to produce new cells in rapid succession (Webster's Dictionary). My definition of prolotherapy as applied medically in the treatment of skeletal disability is "the rehabilitation of an incompetent structure by the generation of new cellular tissue."

A discussion of proliferation solutions, their strength, quantity, frequency and combinations with anesthetic solutions and analgesics will be discussed under Proliferants.

I will endeavor to present as concisely and specifically as possible the technic of procedure in general and for specific ligaments in particular that I have developed and found most effective in the past 19 years so that the reader will be able to carry out the procedure.

Because of the desirability of placing the stimulating solution over as great an area of the fibro-osseous junction as possible and to eliminate multipuncture of the skin, I have developed special technics, particularly for lumbosacral and sacroiliac joint stabilization, that makes possible the injection of a small portion of the solution at from 10 to 15 places against bone from one insertion of the *sharp* needle through the skin.

May I suggest the advisability of refreshing one's memory about the relative position of the ligaments, tendons, and bones by reference to the anatomy.

It is advantageous to frequently familiarize oneself with the skeleton in order to have a three-dimensional picture of the relations of the bones and ligaments. One will be well rewarded to have a spine and pelvis skeleton for office reference.

It may be advantageous for the beginner to first treat the posterior sacroiliac ligament (Fig. 16). It is relaxed more often than any other ligament of the body. It is readily accessible for diagnosis and for needling in confirmation of the diagnosis and in treatment, and it lies in a V-shaped crevice between two bones so it can be readily approached with confidence, and no damage can be done to any other tissue either by needling or by the proliferating solution.

Luerlock, 22-gauge, safety (bead on barrel) needles of sufficient length (1-1½-2-2½-3 inches) are used to distribute the solution at the fibro-osseous junction. If kept sharp by an electric needle sharpener, the needles can be quickly thrust through the skin and inserted the desired length to contact bone with little discomfort. Always tell the patient that you will let him know before you give the treatment, and then just before the insertion through the skin, tell him that there will be a little pain. It will help in relieving apprehension and in keeping him relaxed.

With a sharp needle you will be able to detect the difference in texture of the different layers as encountered by the needle. The denser ligament tissue is readily recognized as well as the abrupt obstruction of the needle by bone while making only light pressure when the tactile sensation of the fingers is more acute.

The beginner may use a syringe containing only an anesthetic solution until he knows the needle is within the ligament and then change syringes to one containing the proliferant.

I am so confident of my diagnosis, the depth of the ligament, and my tactile sensation that I usually only use the proliferant combined with the anesthetic solution and no anesthetic solution alone before entering the ligament or tendon.

Usually the needle is inserted at the trigger point of either ligament or tendon until the point of the needle contacts bone. The local pain is reproduced confirming the diagnosis. The proliferating solution is injected while the point of the needle is held against the bone. If an area of relaxation larger than one inch has been previously determined by palpation, the point of the needle may be changed without withdrawing it from the skin.

If the ligament is thick, some of the solution is distributed as the needle is withdrawn through it.

In areas like the occipital ridge, scapularis muscles, and ribs, the injected area may be massaged with pressure after the needle has been withdrawn to increase the distribution.

Some of the solution may follow the needle channel to the skin. I usually massage each needled area to close the channel.

With the above technic the proliferant is distributed at the fibro-osseous junction where relaxation chiefly takes place and where the new fibrous tissue and bone are desired.

It must always be remembered that the amount of discomfort on injecting solutions depends on the sharpness of the needle and on the slowness with which the solution is injected.

Cervical and Upper Dorsal Spine: For treatment of the articular ligaments of the cervical and upper dorsal spine and the tendon attachments at the occipital line of the skull, scapula and upper ribs, the patient sits astride a chair with his forehead resting on his forearms which are crossed on the back of the chair (Fig. 12). The treatment may be given with the patient in a semiprone position with pillows under his chest, his chin extending just over the pillows, his forehead resting on the table.

The examiner places his left thumb and index finger astride the supraspinus ligament between the cervical spines at the desired level. A 1-inch needle attached to a 10 cc. syringe is inserted through the skin at the desired level and enters the supraspinus and interspinus ligaments. Four cubic centimeters of the proliferating solution is distributed within the ligaments. If the point of the needle contacts bone after piercing the ligaments, some of the solution is injected against the bone before changing position. It will be found that throughout the entire spine there is usually very little relaxation of the supraspinus ligament, and it will be so dense that often none of the solution can be injected until the needle enters the interspinus ligament where relaxation chiefly occurs to account for most of the vertebral articular instability, including many cases of spondylolisthesis with disc compression which is an etiological factor preceding ruptured disc, as described by Alpers.

Before removing the needle from the interspinus ligament, the thumb and index finger are placed astride the adjoining supraspinus ligament for the injection of the interspinus ligament in that space. By this procedure the location does not become confused by movable skin.

When the patient has complained of more pain to one side of the midline and particularly when there is accompanying referred pain into the head, shoulder and upper extremity, a 2-inch needle can be used instead of the 1-inch. Care is used to avoid inserting it more than half its length when injecting the interspinus lingament. The needle is then partly withdrawn until the point is just beneath the skin. It is directed outward at an angle of 30 degrees, and at about its full length, the point will contact bone. The injection of 2 cubic centimeters of the solution is injected into the spinus articular capsular ligament. An injection is also made on the other side if the symptoms and examination so indicate.

In the lower cervical and dorsal interspinus ligaments, a 1½-inch needle is used, and the needle is directed upward at an angle as indicated by the direction of the spines on the skeleton. Approximately 5 to 6 cubic centimeters of the solution is injected.

In the *dorsal area* there is sometimes a trigger point of pain about 1 to 2 inches lateral to the midline due to tendon relaxation at the muscle attachment to the inner end of a rib which can be treated by injection into the trigger point area with the patient in the prone position.

When the tendon attachments to the dorsal surface of the ribs is more than 2 inches in length, it usually requires two insertions of the needle to treat the area because of the difficulty of knowing that the point of the needle is in contact with the rib when the angle of the needle becomes far from the vertical position. Three to five cubic centimeters of proliferant are injected.

Low Back: It is surprising that the preponderance of low back articular ligament relaxation cases completely respond to treatment to their satisfaction, although the x-rays sometimes reveal arthritis, congenital and acquired deformities, degenerations, apparent slight displacements, and disc narrowing.

The *lumbar interspinus ligaments* are treated by the same technic as in the neck with the thumb and index finger astride the supraspinus ligament between the spines of the vertebrae, with the patient in the prone position (Fig. 15). A pillow placed transversely under the abdomen will straighten out the lumbar spine while separating the spines to more readily facilitate the insertion of the needle vertically. A 1½-inch needle is used, but in patients of slight build, the needle is not inserted its full length in the center between the spines, particularly in the lumbosacral space. While directing the needle at an angle to the base of the spines above and below, the full length can be used advantageously. Five to six cubic centimeters of the proliferant solution is injected.

For treatment of relaxation of the *sacrospinalis tendon* attachments to the transverse processes of the lumbar vertebrae, the tip of the left index finger is placed in the interspinus depression, and a 2 to 2½ inch needle is inserted vertically at a point 1-inch lateral to the tip of the finger. At a depth of approximately 1½ inches the point of the needle will contact bone. A total of 5 cubic centimeters is distributed against the process and spine of the vertebra. The opposite side is injected when desired while the location is known before proceeding to a higher or lower vertebra, the tip of the finger being placed in the interspinus depression before the needle is withdrawn from the opposite side. It is frequently advisable to treat a process or two above the highest one which had trigger point tenderness, because the point of the needle and a few drops of the solution will more definitely reproduce the local pain than the tactile pressure of the thumb.

An important *technic* for inserting the needle for both the *iliolumbar* and upper *posterior sacroiliac ligament* is to place the tip of the left index finger in the lumbosacral depression (Fig. 14, O, Fig. 1, LS). The point for inserting the 2½-inch needle vertically downward to the transverse process of the 5th lumbar vertebra is located 1-inch lateral to the top of the finger tip (Fig. 1, 1L, 1). I contact all the lumbar transverse processes nine times out of ten on the initial insertion of the needle. If it is missed, a change in position up or down will contact it. A view of the x-rays will often reveal a short or angled process which will assist in directing the needle. The point for inserting the 3-inch needle into the upper portion of the posterior sacroiliac ligament is ½ inch below the finger and ½ inch from the midline. The needle is directed outward at an angle of 45 degrees and slightly upward (Fig. 1, SI, High, 1).

At each insertion of the needle throughout the skeleton, there is a special point for placing either the thumb or index finger of the left hand to facilitate location of the trigger point area or a bony landmark and for retracting soft tissue, particularly the buttocks.

Treatment of the *iliolumbar ligament* (Fig. 1, IL) includes its attachment to the 5th and usually the transverse process of the 4th lumbar verebra (when 4th lumbar instability is also present); also its attachment to the ilium, the spinus articular capsular ligament and the interlaced group of ligaments that fill the space between the 5th transverse process, the ilium and the top of the sacrum, including the upper sacroiliac notch.

The amount of proliferant solution to cover this area will be approximately 12 cubic centimeters, and it will be distributed at approximately 12 contacts with bone (transverse process of the 5th lumbar vertebra, the anterior surface of the ilium beneath the crest, the top of the sacrum, and the articular processes of the lumbosacral articulation) from one insertion of the needle (Fig. 1, IL, 1). After the needle has contacted the transverse process (Fig. 1, IL, Needle # 1) at two or three places, it is redirected outward and more superficial until it contacts the anterior surface of the ilium (Needle # 2) and redirected further outward and injections made as long as bone or dense ligament tissue is contacted. The needle is then directed into the sacroiliac notch (Needle # 3) and at perhaps three points on top of the sacrum (Needle # 4) and then more superficial to the dorsal surface of the sacrum (Needle # 5) at the articulation of the 5th lumbar and 1st sacral spines.

The injections are made while the needle is in contact with the bone at all places, but it is also made for a short distance as the needle is withdrawn through the ligament at the ilial and sacral attachments where the ligament is thicker, but not on the transverse processes.

At every contact with bone the patient will be aware of the needle being in the right place. Adopt a technic which will perceive light contact with bone, for it is here the sensory nerve supply is most abundant.

When the examination has revealed trigger point tenderness of the 4th lumbar vertebrae interspinus ligament, it is advisable to treat the iliolumbar ligament attachment to the 4th transverse process in the same way as the 5th.

In severe or even moderately severe cases of lumbosacral instability, there is almost invariably an accompanying relaxation of the upper portion of the posterior sacroiliac ligament (Fig. 1, A), and satisfactory results will not be obtained unless both articulations are stabilized.

Treatment of *posterior sacroiliac ligament* relaxation is made with two insertions of the needle. As previously described, a 3-inch needle is inserted at a point ½ inch below the tip of the left index finger in the lumbosacral depression and ½ inch from the midline (Fig. 1, SI, High). Twelve cubic centimeters of the proliferant is injected through this one insertion of the needle at approximately 12 contacts with bone surrounding the upper portion of the sacroiliac joint, except above the articulation in the upper sacroiliac notch and in the space beneath the posterior superior spine of the ilium, where the needle is inserted its full length without contacting bone. Some of the solution is also injected as the needle is withdrawn from contact with the bone at each place.

It is necessary to use the 3-inch needle to reach those upper ligament fibers (Fig. 1, A) from which the referred pain on the outer anterior thigh to above the patella has its origin.

The needle is directed outward at an angle of 45 degrees and slightly upward (Fig. 1, SI, High, 1). I aim to contact bone at the upper margin of the sacroiliac joint, then redirect it higher to avoid bone and insert it the full length. By partial withdrawal

and redirection the point of the needle contacts the upper inner
joint margin, (vertically into the spinus articular capsular ligament if there is accompanying lumbosacral instability), medial
to the sacroiliac joint margin (Fig. 1, SI, High, 2), and beneath
the posterior superior spine (Fig. 1, SI, High, 3), and the full
length of the needle to just below the spine. To get beneath the
spine it will be necessary to withdraw the needle until the point
is just beneath the skin because the sacrum lies much more superficial at that point.

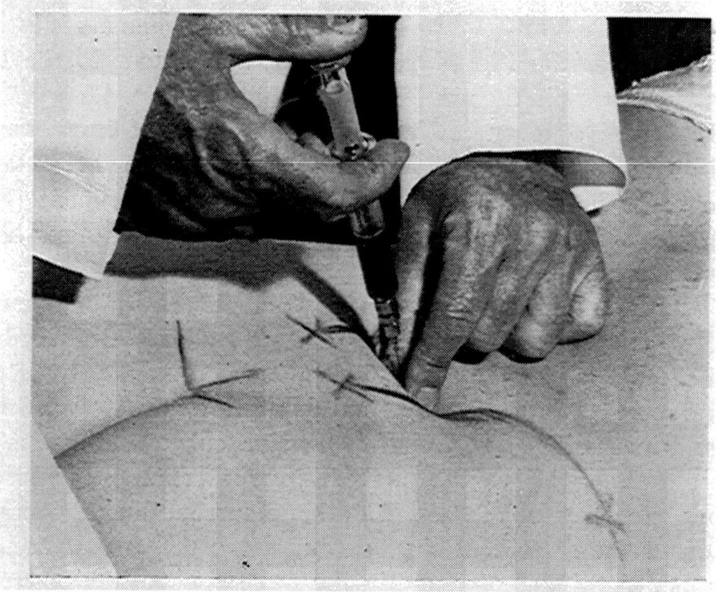

Fig. 15. Patient reclining relaxed for confirmation of the diagnosis and treatment of lower dorsal, lumbar and pelvic ligaments.
Left thumb and finger astride lumbosacral (5th lumbar) supraspinus ligament for insertion of needle into lumbosacral interspinus ligament.

Sometimes even at a second treatment the sacroiliac joint is
so markedly separated that the needle will enter the joint two
or three times, at which time the patient will usually but not
always experience an acute pain. The needle is withdrawn and
slightly redirected against the bone before any of the solution is
injected.

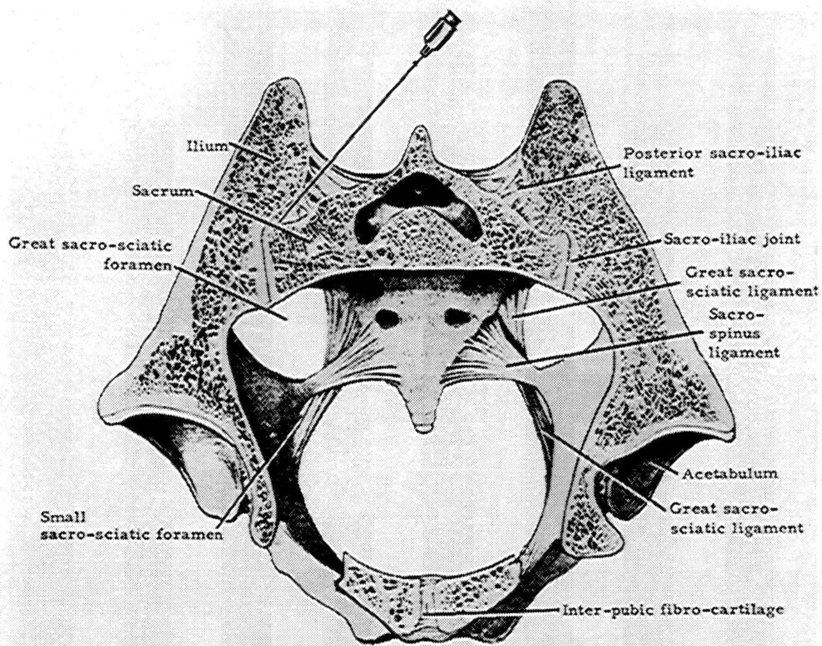

Fig. 16. Transverse section through sacroiliac joints with needle in position of full insertion to joint margin of posterior sacroiliac ligament.

For treating the lower portion of the posterior sacroiliac ligament (Fig. 1, C, D), the left thumb is wiggled into the lower sacroiliac notch just lateral to the posterior superior spine of the ilium (Fig. 1, SI, Low), and a 2½-inch needle is inserted medial to the thumb into the ligaments as it crosses the notch, and into the ligament below the posterior superior spine (Fig. 1, SI, Low, 1), and also under the spine and sometimes the ligament medial to the lower portion of the sacroiliac articulation by changing position of the needle. Partially withdrawing the needle, the point is directed further outward to contact bone underneath the ligament at its attachment to the margin and outer surface of the ilium (Fig. 1, SI, Low, 2) just above the sciatic foramen. A portion of the solution is injected at different bone contacts but only while the point of the needle is in contact with bone, because the sciatic nerve emerges from the pelvis just beneath the ligament. Probably some of the proliferant is injected into the portion of the piriformis tendon which also has some attachment at this point.

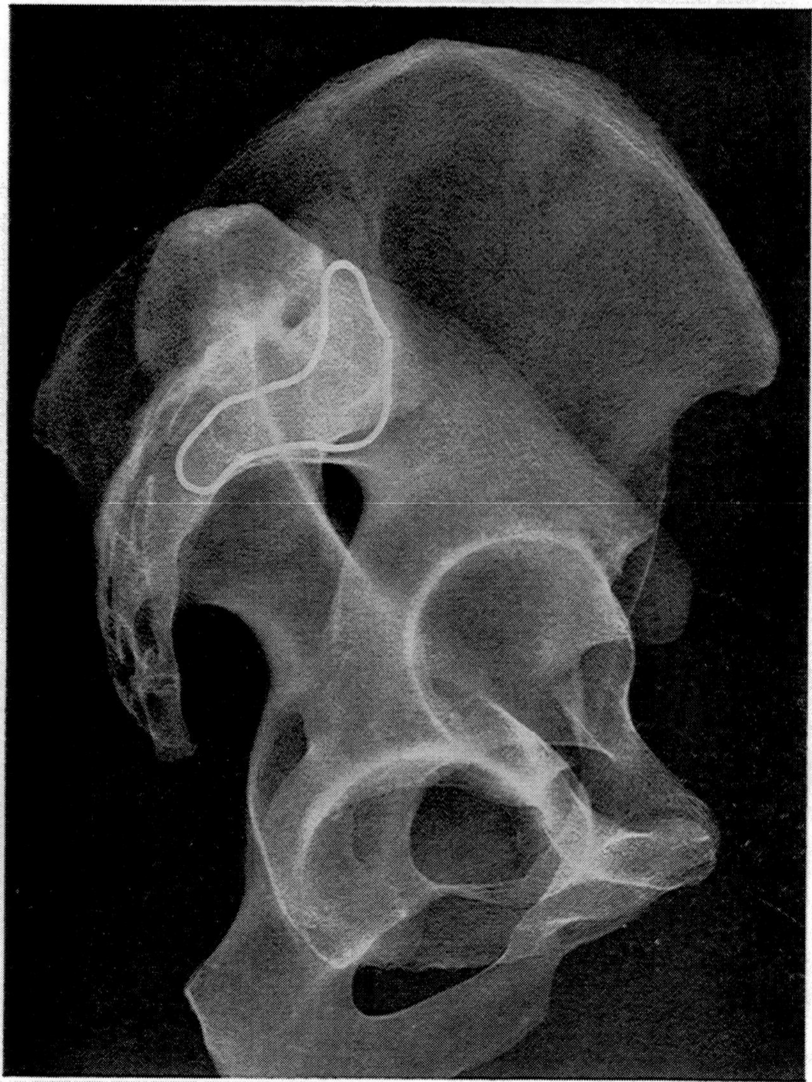

Fig. 17. Roentgenogram of the pelvis in which a wire surrounds the margin of the sacroiliac joint.

Compared with Figure 1, the small joint area emphasizes the importance of the sacroiliac, sacrospinus and sacrotuberus ligaments which have developed during centuries to cover considerable areas in strategic positions, to maintain stability of the articulation.

The lower half of the sacrum extends below the sacroiliac joint and is supported only by ligaments.

(From *Medical Radiography and Photography*. Courtesy C. F. Bridgman and W. S. Cornwell, Eastman Kodak Company, Rochester, New York.)

The needle is then redirected to the outer edge and adjacent dorsal area of the sacrum (Fig. 1, SI, Low, 3) to inject the sacral attachment of the posterior sacroiliac ligament and the sacrospinus and sacrotuberus ligaments (Fig. 1, SS, ST) which are interlaced with it. With this one insertion of the needle, 12 cubic

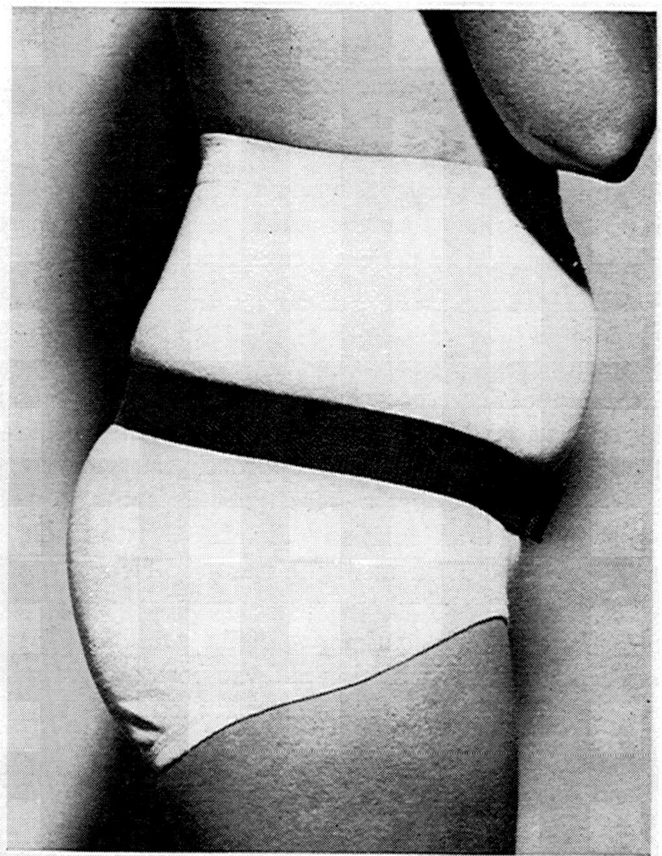

Fig. 18. "Man's belt" (1¼-inch wide such as regular Army belt) binds sacroiliac joints together.

Compare with Figure 16. The belt approximates the two ilium bones posteriorly against the sacrum and relieves strain on the posterior sacroiliac ligaments. It is the best sarcoiliac belt in the world.

Applied at the pubic level, it relieves all patients with unstable sacroiliac joints. If worn for six weeks after treatment, the sacroiliac ligaments will heal stronger without strain.

centimeters of the proliferant is injected, all of it while the needle is held against bone except beneath the posterior spine.

Treatment of relaxation of the *sacrospinus and sacrotuberus* ligaments at their attachments to the sacrum is made by pressing the buttock downward and outward away from the edge of the sacrum halfway between the lower sacroiliac groove and the lower margin of the sacrum, and inserting a 2-inch needle at that point (Fig. 1, SS, ST). Six cubic centimeters of the proliferant is injected in the area along the edge and dorsal surface of the sacrum, between the sacrococcygeal joint and the area on the sacrum which was injected by the low sacroiliac injection. These ligaments must be injected in severe relaxation of the lower portion of the posterior sacroiliac ligament and especially when sciatica is present. Otherwise, the patient's condition will show little improvement. In severe cases of sacroiliac joint instability accompanied by sciatica, the patient will probably require more than one treatment.

Treatment of Sacrococcygeal Ligament. The buttocks is considerably elevated while lying on his abdomen, so the thighs should be flexed to give a better approach by placing a pillow beneath the pelvis. Using a 1-inch needle the area posterior to the sacrococcygeal articulation (Fig. 1, SC) is infiltrated with a local anesthetic solution until the needle pierces the posterior sacrococcygeal ligament and enters the articulation. A syringe is substituted, and 4 cubic centimeters of the proliferating solution is injected within the articulation and the posterior articular ligament. Not more than three treatments at monthly intervals have ever been given to effect a cure; sometimes only one. During the convalescent period, the patient should avoid sitting on any uncomfortable chair, such as an upholstered one, in which the ischial tuberosities sink in and force the material up against the coccyx. A flat wooden (kitchen) chair is best. I have not found it advisable nor necessary to remove a coccyx in 19 years (Case #19).

Treatment of Hip Articular Ligament: The patient lies on the abdomen with the extremity rotated inward. The buttocks is pressed inward with the left thumb close to the upper trochanter of the femur at the trigger point 1-inch below the upper end. A 2½-inch needle is inserted vertically close to the femur (Fig. 1, H) until the point contacts the femur and reproduces the local pain. Six cubic centimeters of the proliferation solution is distributed within the ligament attachments to the femur and ilium by redirecting the needle. Usually benefit and often a satisfactory cure may be accomplished by one to four treatments (Case #20). The hip, however, is the most unsatisfactory articulation that I have treated. I avoid treatment if any substantial amount of arthritis is present and discontinue treatment if there is no benefit after a second treatment.

Acromio-clavicular Joint: Relaxation of the superior acromio-clavicular ligament is accompanied by trigger point pain on top of the articulation. The treatment is by inserting a 1-inch needle transversely within the joint anteriorly (Fig. 19). A local anesthetic is injected in the joint area until the point of the needle enters the articular cavity. The syringe is substituted, and 5 cubic centimeters of the proliferating solution is injected within the joint. The treatment may be repeated in one month. The results are very satisfactory. I have never found it necessary to inject the coraco-clavicular ligament which lies below the clavicle; however, it might be necessary in a more extensive relaxation than I have encountered.

Proximal Radio-ulnar Joint (Elbow): Relaxation of the orbicular ligament (Tennis Elbow) results usually from a continued strain on the ligament in an action that involves rotation of the forearm. It may have begun following a contusion.

The chief symptom is pain on activity involving rotation of the forearm.

There is trigger point tenderness at a particular "spot" which can readily be located by palpation.

The treatment in persistant cases consists in locating the trigger point pain with the tip of the left thumb and inserting a 22-gauge needle past the thumbnail (Fig. 20) until the point of the needle impinges on the bone. One-half cubic centimeter of the proliferant solution is infiltrated into the fibro-osseous junction. Two or three treatments at monthly intervals will suffice for recovery.

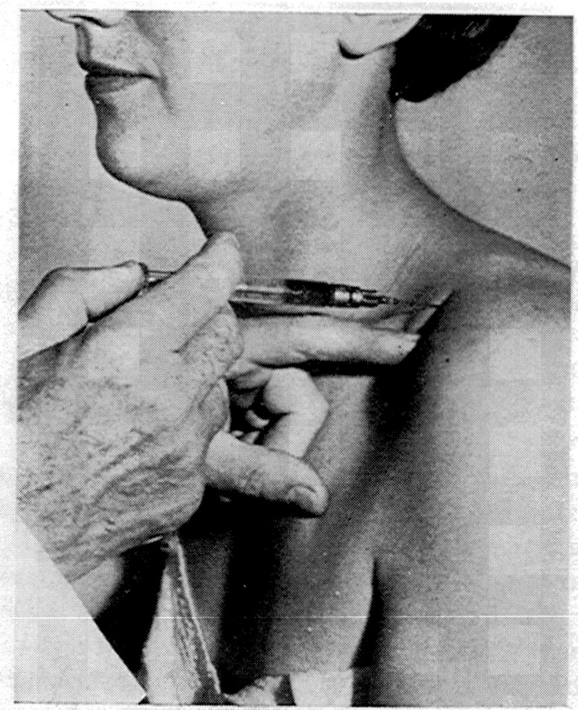

Fig. 19.   Acromio-clavicular joint
Direction of needle for insertion in ligaments and
joint space.

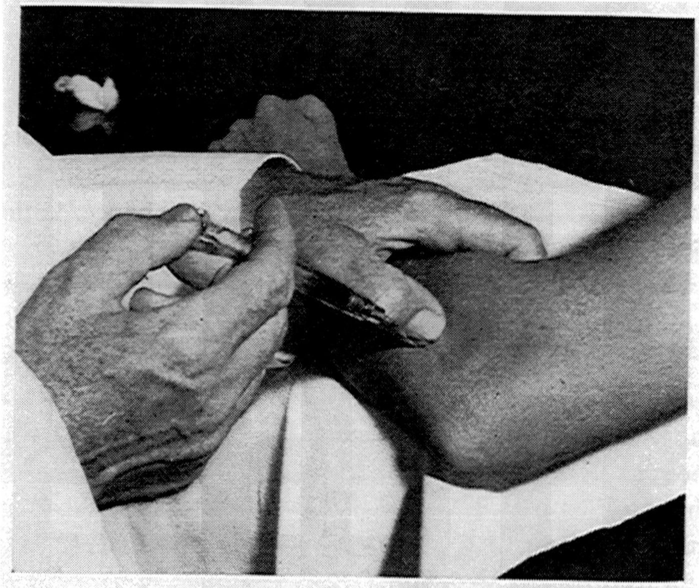

Fig. 20.   Elbow.   Needle in position at "trigger point" in
"Tennis Elbow."

Aggravating activity should be avoided as far as possible during the proliferation period of a few weeks.

There may be accompanying tendon relaxation which will become stabilized by the treatment.

Wrist Joint: Ligament relaxation of the wrist often occurs in that portion of the dorsal ligament that extends from the dorsal surface of the radius to the dorsal surface of the 2nd and 3rd metacarpal bones (Fig. 21). It crosses the scaphoid (navicular), lunate,

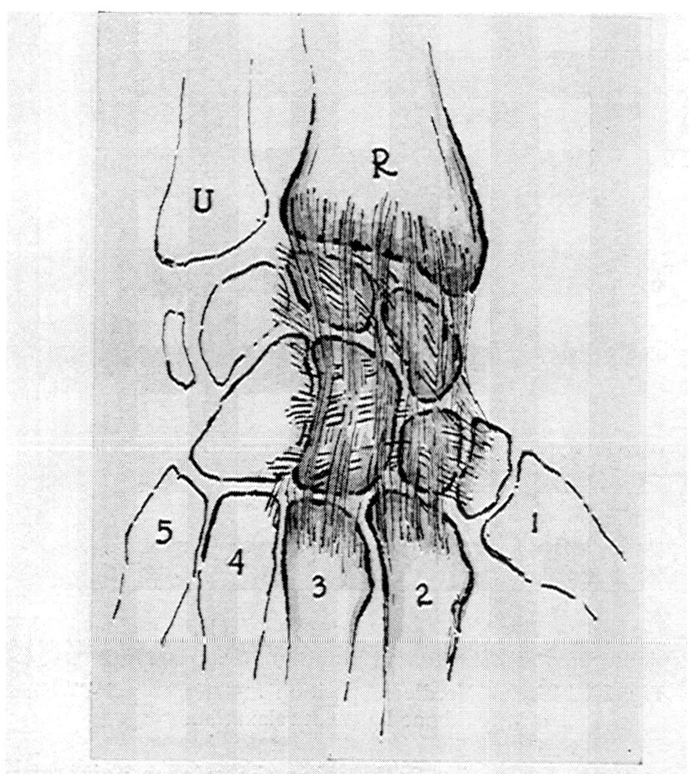

Fig. 21. Wrist. Dorsal ligament between radius—
2nd and 3rd metacarpals, passing over scaphoid,
lunar, trapezoid and capatellum bones.

capitate, and trapezoid bones. It may become relaxed at its attachment to any one of them. Usually there is a history of trauma when the wrist was in extreme flexion.

The pain is severe and recurs frequently during activity which is then necessarily curtailed.

The diagnosis is made by pressing the thumb against the dorsal surface of the carpal bones while the wrist is gently flexed. A sharp referred pain has been observed in a small area just posterior to the acromio-clavicular joint, and it has been reproduced on needling.

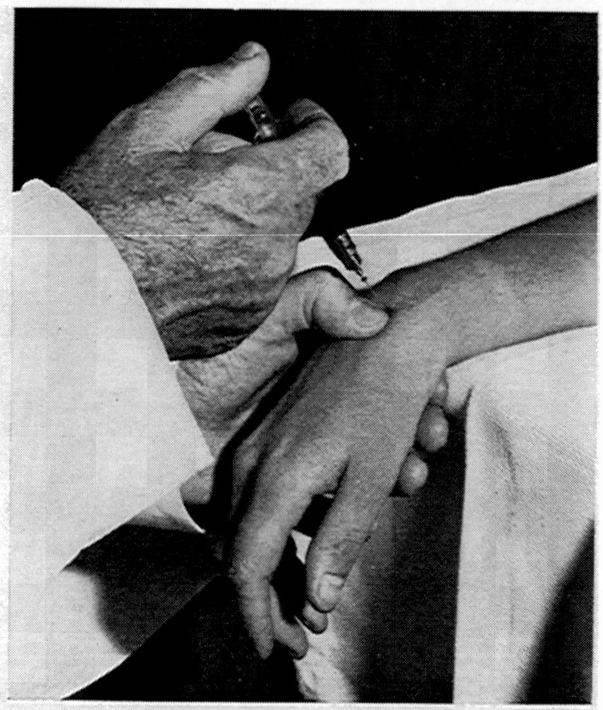

Fig. 22.   Wrist.   Needle in position at "trigger point" of carpal bone ligament relaxation.

The treatment consists in locating the trigger point of pain with the tip of the left thumb while the left fingers gently grasp the wrist which is flexed over the edge of the table. A 22-gauge needle is inserted through the skin at the edge of the thumbnail (Fig. 22). The point of the needle is held against the bone while one-half cubic centimeter of the proliferant solution is injected underneath the ligament at the fibro-osseous junction.

Usually two or three treatments at monthly intervals will provide complete recovery (Case #21).

Ankle Joint: Relaxation of the external lateral ligament ("weak ankle") results from sprains and tearing of the ligament at its attachments to the external malleolus of the fibula. The weakness makes it more susceptible to recurrences and "falls." The ligament is made up of two main bands (Fig. 23). One extends anteriorly to be attached to the talus (#1), while the one which extends downward is attached to the calcaneum (#2).

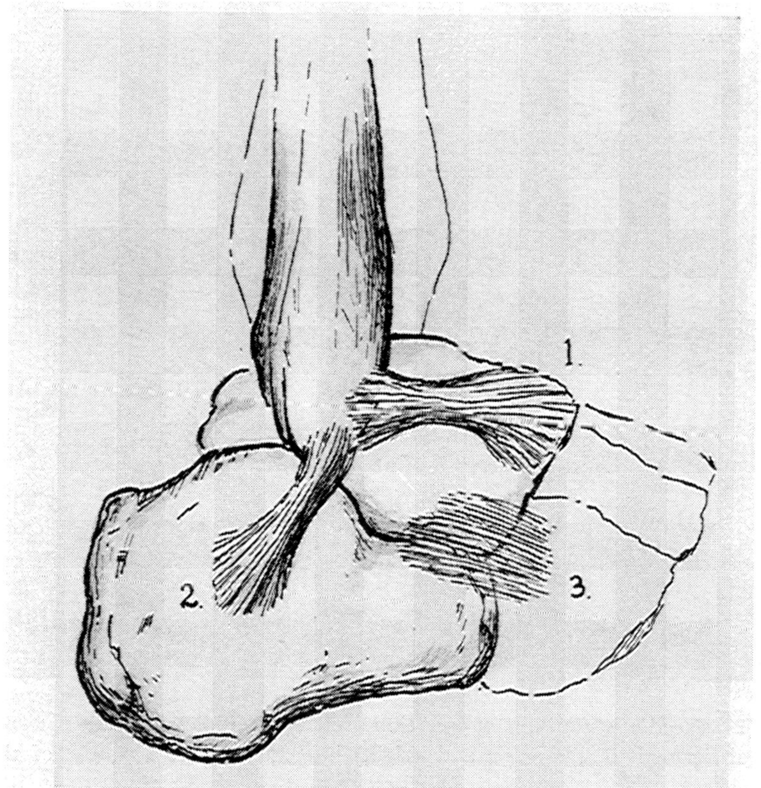

Fig. 23. (1-2) External lateral ligament of ankle. (3) Calcaneo-cuboid ligament of foot.

The relaxation usually occurs at the fibular attachments because of the smaller amount of surface at the fibro-osseous junction.

The trigger point of pain is at the fibular attachment.

The technic of treatment consists of having the medial side of the foot lying on a pillow. The proliferant solution is injected at the malleolar attachment (Fig. 24) by passing one needle attached to a syringe diagonally upward through the ligament at the anterior-inferior margin of the malleolus, while the other needle is passed transversely through the other portion of the ligament at its attachment to the tip of the malleolus.

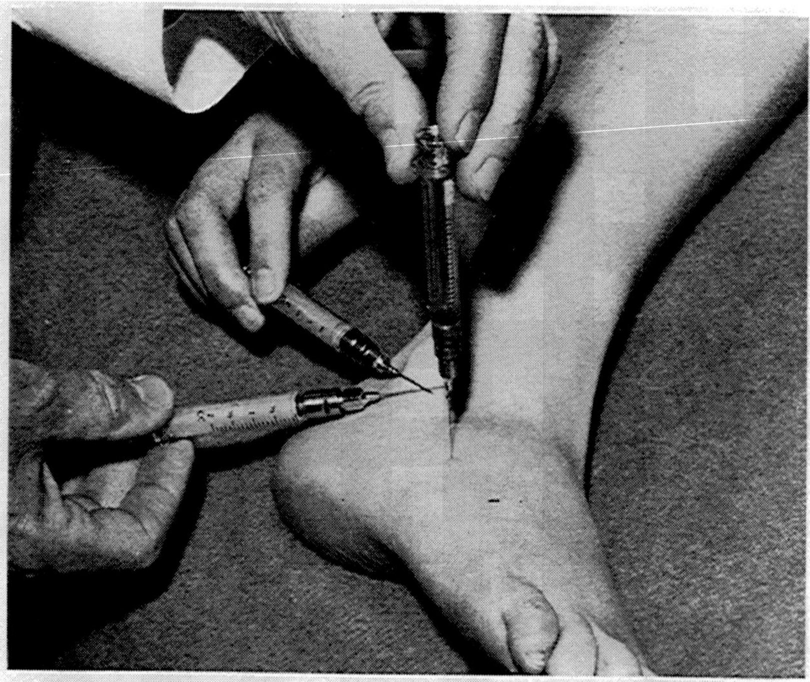

Fig. 24. Needle in position of insertion (left and middle) into the external lateral ligament of the ankle and (right) into an articular ligament of the foot.

One-half cubic centimeter of the proliferant solution is distributed through each tibial attachment at one office call. Two or three treatments are usually required for each portion of the ligament at monthly intervals.

An elastic ankle brace may be worn during the convalescent period to add comfort and to prevent stretching of the ligament during the stabilization period (Case #22).

Foot: Various ligaments of the foot become relaxed. One that I have successfully treated is the calcaneo-cuboid together with the strands attached between the astragalus and the cuboid (Fig. 23).

The trigger point of fibro-osseous relaxation is located by palpation with the finger.

Treatment consists of the injection of one-half cubic centimeter of the proliferating solution beneath the ligament at the trigger point area while the point of the needle is held against the bone (Fig. 24). One or two treatments are usually sufficient.

On one occasion when I had removed a bone spur from the inferior medial surface of the distal end of the 1st metatarsal bone, I injected the proliferating solution throughout a relaxed painful transverse metatarsal ligament. The patient made an excellent recovery which resulted in a painless walking foot. I do not know how much benefit to attribute to the injection, but I firmly believe the treatment of the extremities by fibro-osseous proliferation will be greatly extended when other investigators undertake it.

Tendon Relaxation

Any tendon throughout the body may become chronically relaxed and the origin of pain.

In different sections of the body, there are some tendons that become relaxed more often than others. I will discuss the ones that I have most frequently encountered.

Figure 25 and Figure 26-1 reveal the trigger points of tendons attached to the *occipital* bone. They are the tendons of the upper back muscles that are used in movements of the head and are subject to a great deal of tension and trauma. They are often injured along with the ligaments of the neck and together are the most common cause of the so-called "whiplash" injuries.

Most of the headache that originates in the occipital area with referred pain up over the head has its origin in these relaxed occipital tendons.

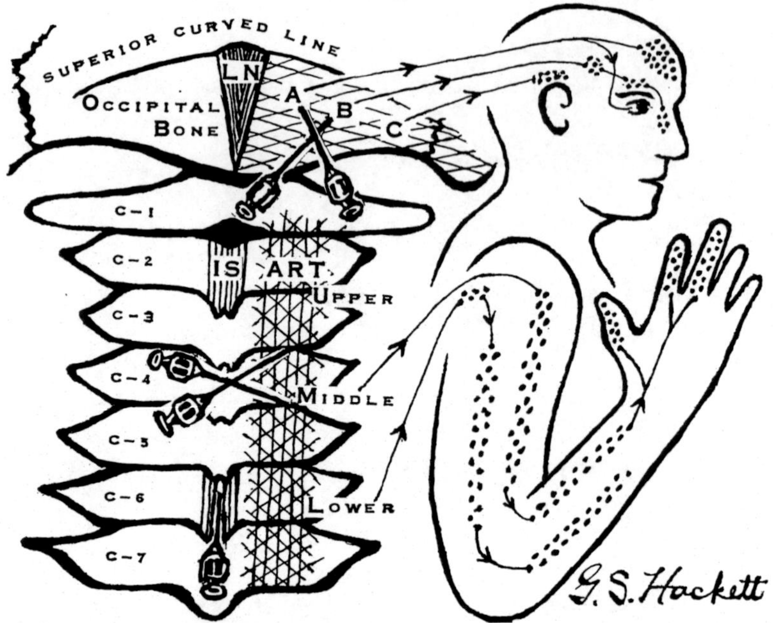

TRIGGER POINTS — REFERRED PAIN AREAS
POSITION OF NEEDLES FOR DIAGNOSIS AND TREATMENT

OCCIPITAL TENDONS
REFERRED PAIN, HEADACHE, DIZZINESS
A – FOREHEAD, EYE
B – TEMPLE, EYEBROW, NOSE
C – ABOVE EAR

CERVICAL LIGAMENTS
IS — INTERSPINUS LIGAMENTS
ART —ARTICULAR LIGAMENTS
REFERRED PAIN
UPPER – NECK
MIDDLE – ARM, FOREARM, THUMB,
1 AND 2 FINGERS
LOWER – ACROMIUM PROCESS, ARM,
FOREARM.

Fig. 25.

The tendon attachment at Figure 25-A has a referred pain to the forehead and into the eye. From Figure 25-B the referred pain extends into the temple and nose. From Figure 25-C the referred pain extends up over the ear, and from Figure 25-D there is headache associated with loss of equilibrium on movements of the head, particularly on raising the head after stooping.

These referred pains have been reproduced by needling and often clear up permanently after the first treatment, although it may take two treatments to permanently eliminate the local pain and headache. The positions and directions of the needles are illustrated in Figure 25. In making these injections the patient is placed on his abdomen. Two pillows are placed lengthwise beneath the chest so that the flexed neck will permit the chin to rest against the end of the pillow while the forehead resting on the table will straighten out the lordotic curve of the neck and facilitate the approach with the needles to both the occipital tendons and the cervical ligaments and tendons.

The attachment of the ligamentum nuchae (Fig. 25-LN) may become relaxed with a referred pain centrally in the occipital region.

The cervical articular ligaments (Figs. 25-ART, 26-2) are attached to the posterior surface of the lamina and transverse processes of the cervical vertebrae and have a referred pain from the upper cervical vertebra extending to the side of the neck. From the middle section of the cervical vertebrae, the referred pains extend into the arm, forearm, thumb, first and second fingers. From the lower cervical articular ligaments, the referred pain extends to the clavicular area just posterior to the acromial process, antero-lateral arm and forearm.

A 2-2½ inch needle directed outward from the midline at a 30 degree angle will reproduce the local pain on encountering bone and sometimes the referred pain. There is frequently an accompanying tendon relaxation of the cervical muscles which are attached to the articular ligaments in the cervical as well as the dorsal and lumbar articular ligaments so that when the trigger point pain is reproduced and treatment given, the solution penetrates both ligaments and tendons, and proliferation ensues in both.

The trigger points of the occipital tendons are easily located by having the patient first locate the tender "spot." The relaxed articular ligaments and their overlying relaxed tendons throughout the spine are located by pressure lateral to the transverse processes and the pain reproduced by needling.

There is no hazard in injecting the occipital area because the point of the needle is against bone while the injection is made. There is also no hazard in injecting the articular tendons and ligaments in the cervical area because the point of the needle impinges on bone at every point of the injection. Also the important nerves and blood vessels lie anterior to the lamina and transverse processes. Only above the third cervical vertebra could the needle miss bone and be directed too deeply. Below the third vertebra there is no space between the lamina through which a needle could pass if it is directed transversely at a 30 degree angle and not directed upward.

Tendon Relaxation Trigger Points—Figure 26

Figure 26: (1) Represents the trigger points of tendon attachment to the occipital bone.

(2) Represents the trigger points of tendon attachments to the cervical vertebrae as described above (also articular ligaments).

(3) Represents tendon attachments to the dorsal spine, articular ligaments, and the angle of the rib.

(4) Represents the tendon attachments to the spines, articular ligaments, and the transverse processes of the lumbar vertebrae.

(5) Represents the sacrospinalis tendons attached to the sacrum and the posterior sacroiliac ligament.

(6) Represents the gluteus maximus tendons attached to the sacrum and the posterior sacroiliac ligaments.

(7) Represents the upper ribs to which a variety of tendons are attached. The most common complaint is found in patients with poor posture in a stooped position or who work in that position. They are the persons who get relief by throwing back their head and shoulders. The tender painful areas are usually more extensive like a muscle fatigue soreness than the trigger points of tendon relaxation. The postural strain on the muscles from

TENDON RELAXATION

TRIGGER POINTS

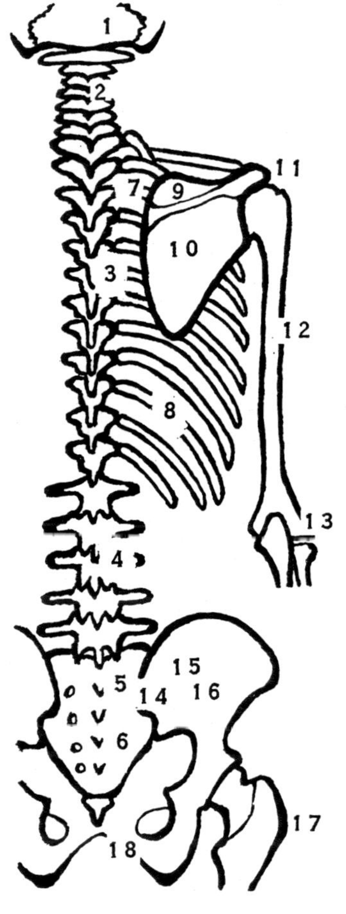

1 OCCIPITAL .

2 CERVICAL VERTEBRA .

3 DORSAL VERTEBRA .

4 LUMBAR VERTEBRA .

5 SACRUM. SACROSPINALIS.

6 SACRUM. GLUTEUS MAXIMUS

7 RIBS. POSTURAL STRAIN.

8 RIBS. ILIOCOSTALIS, ETC.

9 SCAPULA. SUPRASPINATUS

10 SCAPULA. INFRASPINATUS.

11 SCAPULA. DELTOID ORIGIN.

12 HUMERUS. DELTOID INS.

13 HUMERUS. LAT. EPICONDYLE.

14 ILIUM. GLUTEUS MAXIMUS.

15 ILIUM. GLUTEUS MEDIUS.

16 ILIUM. GLUTEUS MINIMUS.

17 FEMUR. GT. TROCHANTER.

18 PUBES. DESCENDING RAMUS.

Fig. 26.

stretching and sustained contractions produce noxious metabolites which results in spasm or "cramp." This in turn engenders pain by excessive traction on the nerves at the fibro-osseous junction followed by a reflex arteriospasm and ischemia of the muscle. The change of posture quickly relieves the discomfort. Sometimes it is necessary to inject a proliferant at the tendon attachment to the upper four ribs, but more often a satisfactory method is to explain about posture and have the patient fitted with the Camp shoulder brace, Model 53 as shown in Figure 31. Advise them to wear it until relief is obtained and to replace it as a reminder whenever the pain reappears.

(8) Represents the trigger points of iliocostalis tendon relaxation that occurs along the dorsal surface of the ribs from 3 to 5 inches in length. The length of the trigger point areas are easily determined. The treatment by prolotherapy is successful. Referred pain along the course of the accompanying nerve which may extend to the midline anteriorly usually has its origin at the articular ligament and tendons rather than from relaxed tendons along the rib some distance from the spine.

(9) Represents the trigger point of relaxed supraspinatus tendons and (10) represents the infraspinatus tendon trigger point. The trigger point areas vary considerably in size, are easily outlined and treated (Case #30).

(11) Represents the trigger point of relaxed deltoid tendon attachment to the outer edge of the acromial process of the scapula and the "rotator cuff" trigger points of the ligament and tendon attachments at the anatomical neck of the humerus, while (12) represents the trigger point of the relaxed deltoid tendon insertion into the outer surface of the humerus. It is my opinion that fully half of the so-called "bursitis" cases in the shoulder area are due to tendon relaxation and will respond favorably to Prolotherapy. I have found tendon and capsular ligament relaxation trigger points at the margin of the acromial process and at the rotator cuff in cases that the x-ray reveals calcium deposits. X-ray, cortisone, and other treatments had been ineffectual. They responded promptly to Prolotherapy.

I am getting results in recurrent shoulder dislocation by injecting the ligament/tendon trigger points beneath the acromial process of the scapula posteriorly and at the rotator cuff of the humerus posteriorly.

I believe that further investigation of the cervical and shoulder areas will reveal that tendon and ligament relaxation will account for most of the cases that have been attributed to radiculitis, bursitis, periarthritis, tendonitis, causalgia, and a variety of syndromes such as rotator cuff, shoulder-hand, etc. as well as reflex distrophy, post-traumatic osteoporosis, and spinal root compression from osteoarthritis.

(13) Represents the trigger point of the relaxed pronator tendon attachment to the external condyle of the humerus together with the relaxed articular ligament of the head of the radius which together make up the so-called "tennis elbow" and "radio-humeral bursitis" disability which responds to Prolotherapy.

(14), (15) and (16) Trigger point areas of tendon relaxation of the gluteus maximus (14), gluteus medius (15), and gluteus minimus (16) on the ilium. They have been diagnosed as "herniated fat pads," "panicular hernias," and "fibro-lipomatous nodules." Critical analysis has failed to reveal herniated fat or any abnormal pathological findings. Few surgeons have been encouraged to continue removing the palpated nodules because of the disappointing results. Surgeons with a traumatizing technic probably had better results because of the fibrous tissue proliferation that ensued.

Although I have found the trigger point areas throughout the ilium, the most frequent location is on and above the middle gluteal line on the outer surface of the ilium (15) where the gluteus medius tendon is attached. Next most frequent is on and below the middle gluteal line at the gluteus minimus tendon attachment (16). The gluteus maximus tendon is sometimes relaxed at (14) which is located on the posterior superior spine at the posterior gluteal line and also beneath the outer margin of the crest of the ilium anywhere along the superior gluteal line of attachment to as far as the anterior superior spine. The gluteus minimus relaxation between the anterior superior spine and the rim of the acetabulum has resulted from a fall. The gluteal tendon relaxations may occur without any other low back disability, but it accompanies sacroiliac and lumbrosacral joint ligament relaxation so frequently that I now look for it in every case of low back disability. I have missed it so frequently while treating posterior sacroiliac ligament relaxation because its pain is usually overshadowed by the sacroiliac instability which I have been looking for. It stands out like a sore thumb when the sacroiliac disability has been entirely eliminated.

The gluteal tendon pain may be induced and aggravated by coughing, sneezing, crossing the leg over the knee on the same or opposite side, stooping over, walking, or lying in bed. I have observed referred pain from gluteal tendon relaxation to extend to the foot, posterior to the external malleolus, but the areas of relaxation vary so much that there are no referred pain areas that are useful in diagnosis by directing attention to a specific tendon.

The most useful observation is to have the patient place *one finger* on the spot that is the center of his difficulty, and then have him press hard enough to reproduce the pain. Of course, this *one finger by the patient* location of pain should *always* be used in tendon and ligament examinations throughout the body, otherwise hunting for it by the examiner will often confuse both the patient and the examiner.

Treatment of gluteal tendon relaxation is very successful by Prolotherapy. The proliferating solution is injected only against bone and is distributed throughout the trigger point area which is outlined in extent by palpation and needling.

(17) Represents the trigger point area of the muscle and tendon relaxation on the greater trochanter of the femur which becomes more painful on walking any distance and when lying on it.

(18) Represents trigger point tenderness of the tendons of the adductor muscles of the thigh at their attachment to the descending ramus of the pubic bone. It has a referred pain on the inside of the thigh which may extend to the inside of the calf of the leg accompanied by muscular degeneration of the thigh and calf and a limp. Herpes in the referred pain area have been observed (Case #24).

Relaxation of the rectus tendon at the attachment around the upper and lateral margins of the patella as well as the reflected tendonous fibers to the anterior surface of the tibia lateral to the patella ligament may occur alone or as a complication to relaxation of the crucial or patellar ligaments and when severe will prevent straight-leg raising followed by inactivity, muscular degeneration and decalcification. Prolotherapy at the trigger points on the patella and tibia are successful.

The Achilles tendon may become relaxed at the muscular attachment, but usually the torn fibers become strongly attached if aggravation by walking is avoided.

Posture and obesity are important factors in causing tendon relaxation, particularly by increasing the lordotic curves of the lumbar and cervical vertebrae which tends to pull the muscles away from the concavity of the lordosis together with the additional strain on the muscles to carry the load of obesity.

I have come to believe that tendon relaxation can result from pain. In lumbosacral and sacroiliac ligament relaxation, the muscles endeavor to relieve the pain, until they endure long periods of spastic contraction that actually strain the tendon fibers until they become chronically relaxed and themselves become a source of pain on normal muscle contraction.

Close-Jointed vs. Loose-Jointed

From an osteological consideration individuals are genetically divided into two main classes: the close-jointed and the loose-jointed types.

It is an inherited characteristic in which the proclivity of osteogenesis is the important factor in growth, susceptibility to disability, and recovery from disability.

I have been aware of the variation for some 30 years as to its importance in certain types of injury. From my concentration for many years on articular ligament disability, I have made some observations that I do not believe are generally known. They are valuable in diagnosis and in evaluating the disability.

(Fig. 27) The relationship of thumb-finger-forearm of a close-jointed individual on the left and the loose-jointed individual on the right illustrate a somatic division of humanity that have different characteristics. Just as we have tall and short, fat and thin, hyper- and hypoacidic, and hyper- and hypotensive types, so also do we have the two somatic types.

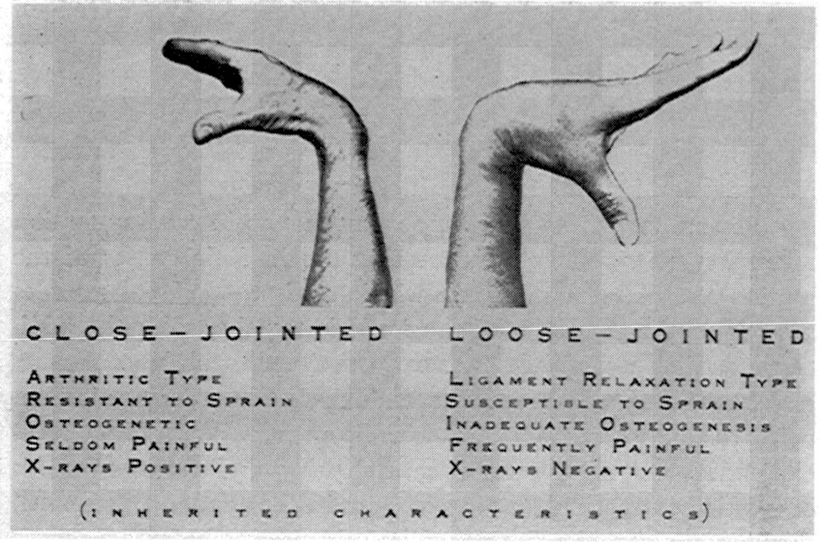

Fig. 27.

In the *close-jointed* type the fingers will not extend beyond a straight line with the metacarpal bones, and when the wrist is fully flexed, the first metacarpal and proximal phalanx of the thumb will not flex beyond a right angle with the radius. The elbow and knee joints will not hyperextend, and the arches of the feet are good.

In the loose-jointed (double-jointed) type on the right in Figure 27 the fingers can be hyperextended, and the thumb can be hyperextended so that in some cases it will touch the forearm. The elbow and knee joints will hyperextend, and the arches of the feet are flat.

The close-jointed type has a proclivity of osteogenesis so that during the growth period he will develop an abundant fibro-osseous attachment of ligaments and tendons to bone so that they will be more resistant to ordinary strain. Following an injury to the fibro-osseous attachment or fractures, he will physiologically make osteoblastic repair to a greater extent than the loose-jointed type.

The close-jointed type is more susceptible to arthritic deposits of calcium, and the joints may be completely bridged by calcium deposits in and about the ligaments. This usually develops without pain unless there is a period of acute intense inflammation or an extension involving the articular surface.

The loose-jointed type has the proclivity of osteogenesis to a less degree so that the fibro-osseous attachment of ligaments and tendons to bone are less resistant to strain, and the hyperextension of the joints permits a greater strain to be placed on the comparatively weakened tissue.

Following injury to the ligaments and tendons, the loose-jointed individual does not physiologically repair the fibro-osseous junction adequately in response to somatic sensory stimulation so that ligament and tendon relaxation with accompanying pain more often results than in the close-jointed type.

The proclivity of osteogenesis is probably determined by a combination of inherited characteristics in the internal glandular complex.

Fortunately, both types respond to increased fibro-osteogenesis by the stimulating influence of a proliferant solution when placed in the periosteum.

Both types can be recognized in early childhood, and especially the loose-jointed individuals should be encouraged to participate in a variety of daily work and exercises during the entire growth period so that the fibro-osseous junctions throughout the body will grow strong, like the head-carrying women of the world who never have neck or back disability because they begin gradually at the age of 5 years to work and exercise.

I frequently encounter backs and other portions of the body that break down from ordinary house and garden work and golf after the growing period in individuals who did not actively participate in them earlier.

Few physicians realize in the interpretation of x-rays that a small amount of lipping usually indicates a more substantial joint, for it occurs at the ligamentous attachment to bone.

When my patients give a history of back disability for periods up to 65 years' duration and negative x-ray reports, an examination revealing excessive thumb and finger extension will indicate ligament relaxation as the cause of the disability.

Multiple ligaments and tendons may become relaxed in the loose-jointed individual so that a psychosomaticly minded physician will recommend psychoanalysis, because he cannot comprehend a patient having such a variety of painful areas. I have cured patients (Case #23) who had multiple ligament and tendon relaxations from the occiput to the coccyx.

Several Miami student nurses visiting my scientific booth at the Southern Medical Association meeting had low back pain that had its origin since entering nursing school. Each one was loose-jointed and had painless flat feet. They all give a history of having done a considerable amount of walking throughout their growth period, but little if any work or activities that would have strengthened their back ligaments during the growth period. Consequently, their feet ligaments developed sufficient strength to go through life without pain unless they later become obese, while their back ligaments did not develop enough strength to withstand the strain imposed by nurses' training. This is an excellent example of the effect of our mechanized age on the human race.

Subsequent Treatment

Rather than prolong the treatment over several weeks as was done in the earlier years, it is now my procedure to complete all the treatment in from one to three days and have the patient return in 6 to 8 weeks for re-evaluation and additional treatment if necessary. It is not satisfactory in the severe cases that require a considerable number of injections to prolong the discomfort and keep them returning during that period. Many of the patients travel hundreds of miles, some from overseas. The most severe cases are hospitalized for 3 to 10 days. Less severe cases are accommodated in hotels within walking distance and return to the office 1 or 2 days to complete the treatment, and then return home when they desire, preferably by plane which is quicker and more comfortable.

Most cases receive the complete treatment and return home the same day, but more than a hundred miles by automobile the same day is not encouraged because of the discomfort after the local anesthesia wears off.

The reason for delaying re-evaluation 6 to 8 weeks is because the proliferant action apparently builds up new tissue from 4 to 6 weeks, and the patient will be better able to appreciate this improvement and to better evaluate any remaining disability. Also the examining physician can arrive at a better estimate after all reaction has subsided.

Local patients may be given a portion of their injections, return in 2 to 7 days for the remainder, and then return in 6 to 8 weeks for re-evaluation.

Proliferants—Anesthetics

There are two proliferating solutions now in use; one for office treatment, the other for hospitalized patients, although either can be used in the office.

Sylnasol (G. D. Searle & Co., Chicago) is the proliferant which we have used satisfactorily for 19 years. It is a solution of the sodium salt of fatty acids of a vegetable oil, which was selected because it has been found to have the ideal qualities of a proliferant which include the induction of a minimal amount of early exudate and discomfort and later a maximum amount of fibrous tissue and bone which become permanent.

For office treatment, it is combined one part with the local anesthetic solution, Pontocaine, 0.15 per cent (Winthrop Laboratories), three parts, making a 25 per cent proliferant solution.

For the hospitalized patients, the Sylnasol is combined one part with normal saline two parts, making a 33 per cent solution, which apparently stimulates a larger amount of proliferation, and the stronger reaction can be adequately controlled by analgesics in the hospital. Preliminary sedatives at bedtime and two hours before treatment, followed by Demerol solution (Winthrop Laboratories), 150 mg. (equivalent to morphine, $\frac{1}{4}$ grain) one hour before treatment obviates the necessity of combining the proliferant with a local anesthetic, so that a considerable quantity of Sylnasol (practically devoid of toxicity when given within ligaments and tendons) can be given at one time without combining it with a local anesthetic solution which in considerable quantity does have toxic effects.

I have given as much as 50 cubic centimeters of Sylnasol to one patient in a one hour period during a course of treatment in the hospital.

Zinc sulfate is the proliferant which we are now using in the treatment of patients in the office. It is combined with phenol and Pontocaine, and has the advantage of a shorter duration of severe painful reaction following the post-treatment local anesthetic period, if only a *small* amount is injected at each point of the needle against bone.

The severe reaction period to be controlled by strong analgesics is usually about 6 hours.

The reaction of both proliferants can be reduced by using greater dilutions, by smaller injections, and by a fewer number of injections.

We have used the zinc sulfate solution as a proliferant in approximately 700 cases over a period of 18 months in which we have been able to observe its reactions and favorable results. We believe we are getting a more favorable proliferation of new cellular reaction. However, we are unable to give as many treatments in one day as when using Sylnasol, because of the toxicity of Phenol if given in a considerable quantity.

The injections are limited to about ten in one day of 3 cubic centimeters of the solution for each treatment. The solution is of sufficient strength that only *half* the quantity per injection is used as when using Sylnasol. This has the advantage of getting a more concentrated proliferating solution at the fibro-osseous junction than when a weaker 6 cubic centimeter injection is given. An additional ten injections can be given on succeeding days.

The zinc sulfate stock solution can be made up by any chemist. (See Material Used By The Author for the formula.)

Extremely nervous or sensitive patients can be treated under Sodium Pentothal anesthesia in the hospital after the diagnosis has been made and the areas for injection are known. It is appreciated by the patient. I have not had any unfavorable reaction from using general anesthesia, but I much prefer to have the patient able to inform me about the reproduction of the local pain. It is a difficult procedure about the neck with the patient lying on his abdomen.

Pontocaine, 0.15 per cent was selected as the local anesthetic to be combined with the proliferants after many years of search to find a compatibly miscible local anesthetic solution which when combined with the proliferant would have the following features: (1) minimal irritation on contact with ligament; (2) quick acting anesthesia; (3) long lasting anesthesia, and (4) no separation, precipitation or flocculent formation after standing for several weeks. It also has world-wide distribution and is one of the local anesthetic solutions to which there are fewer allergic manifestations.

Some physicians are reporting a too severe and prolonged reaction following the zinc sulfate injections as compared with their experience with Sylnasol. I believe it is due to depositing too much and too strong zinc sulfate in a small area, as I also have observed. It should be remembered that *one treatment* (6 cc. of Sylnasol solution, or 3 cc. of zinc sulfate solution) should be distributed at not less than six needle point areas from one skin insertion of the needle. As many as fifteen treatments have been given at one time in selected cases.

Medication—Aftercare

Most hospital cases have their preliminary examination in the office.

Preliminary medication for hospital cases is a full sedative at bedtime and analgesics if necessary. Full sedative two hours before treatment, and Demerol, 150 mg. (or equivalent to morphine, gr. $\frac{1}{4}$) one hour before treatment.

Following treatment in the hospital, strict orders are given that the patient must be kept comfortable, and before reaction pain becomes severe, full doses of hypodermic analgesics are started, repeated in one hour if necessary, and thereafter as needed. The patients are instructed that they will have a reaction and to ask for "hypos" before the pain becomes severe.

Intravenous glucose and saline is given if the patient is nauseated or not taking adequate fluids, which is necessary. Avoid fruit or fruit juices until taking solid foods. Only tea drinkers should be given tea. Dramimine, 50 mg. is given every 4-6 hours for vomiting. By mouth, the best cure of nausea has always been sipping *boiling* water. It stimulates peristalsis from the throat down and washes out the stomach either up or down. Ginger ale is usually the first liquid to be well tolerated after boiling water.

Remain in bed while nauseated with a receptacle at arms length to avoid arising which accentuates nausea and vomiting. Avoid fruit and juices.

Solid food should not be taken either before or after treatment because the analgesics prevent food absorption.

Bathroom privileges as soon as desired.

A saline laxative two days after treatment is given because of the constipating effect of analgesics. No patient can be made comfortable when toxic from colon absorption.

The patient is discharged from the hospital when he is able to travel comfortably.

Office cases are frequently given 50 mg. of Demerol (1 cc.) intramuscularly preliminary to treatment. They are then instructed to turn over on the abdomen without raising the head to avoid dizziness or nausea.

Following treatment, patients are prescribed thirty tablets of either Demerol, 100 mg., Levo-Dromoran, 2 mg., or codeine, 1 gr. to be taken with two aspirins before any uncomfortable reaction begins. They are to repeat the dose in one hour if uncomfortable and then repeat less often as needed.

A full dose of sedative on arriving home and at bedtime will reduce the sensitivity to pain. There is a great difference in the sensitivity of patients to pain. Some only take one or two tablets. A nauseated patient will not absorb medicine from the intestines. Sipping boiling water will often assist absorption.

Baume Bengué applied to the painful area and heat, preferably by the electric pad, are welcomed by the patient. Some prefer a heat lamp to the electric pad.

As the patients begin to feel better, they must avoid any activity that puts a strain on the ligaments or tendons that have been treated, because the new cells are weak, and the anticipated benefit will be less if the cells are subjected to strain before they become strong, over a 6 weeks' period.

It is best to avoid any movement or activity that reproduces their pain. Do not have any manipulation or exercises.

Patients with extremely severe sacroiliac disability and *all* cases with accompanying sciatica should obtain crutches and not put *any* weight on the affected leg until it can be done without pain. The sacroiliac belt should also be worn day and night.

Garments, lumbosacral belts and braces should be worn for six weeks, adjusted comfortably to limit motion.

A Camp shoulder brace (Model #53) (Fig. 28) should be worn by all upper back cases as long as ligament or tendon pain continues or at least one month. It is also excellent for treating those patients who have a pain in the muscular area between the neck and scapula, which comes on after working in a stooped position. They develop the aching from strain on the tendon attachments of the muscle to bone and are relieved by throwing back their head and shoulders. They should re-apply it as a postural reminder every time the pain re-appears.

A belt such as shown in Figure 18 (U. S. Army) is fitted and given to every sacroiliac disability patient to be worn at the level of the pubic bone. (A "little belly" helps to hold it down.)

Wearing it is delayed a few days after treatment until soreness subsides, and it is worn daily for 6 weeks and longer if additional treatment is necessary.

It is the best type of sacroiliac belt obtainable because it "binds" the sacroiliac joints better than the wider belts that extend over the fleshy folds of the abdomen and buttock and prevents strain on the sacroiliac ligaments during the healing period.

Both men and women should wear it after being cured when they participate in such activities as golf, bowling, gardening, car

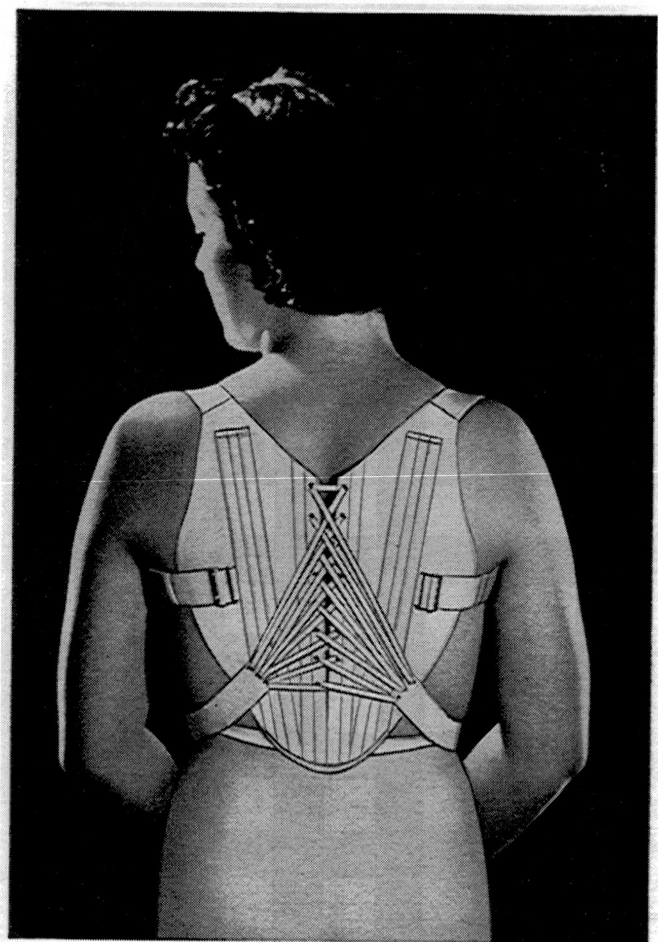

Fig. 28. Camp shoulder brace #53.

I have found this shoulder brace comfortable and efficient in supporting the lower cervical and dorsal spine following Prolotherapy in those areas until the ligaments and tendons were permanently strengthened. Also it is most efficient in correcting posture in those patients whose upper back and neck-shoulder muscles, tendons and ligaments are under strain and ache from poor posture both while sitting and standing.

washing or polishing, painting, scrubbing, sweeping, furniture moving, and fishing.

For 60 years I have observed workmen in many countries wearing their belts over their trousers at this level. It took me 40 years to figure it out. It is diagnostic because it will provide comfort to every sacroiliac patient but to no other condition.

Recently we have been furnishing a more satisfactory belt that does not "cut in" or "slip up." It will not stretch throughout its center, but the edges are elastic to conform to the "bulges" while providing tension. (See "Material Used By The Author" in back of book.)

Debilitated and anemic patients should be built up so they have the capacity to become rehabilitated by producing new bone tissue when treated. Vitamins and estrogens are frequently needed.

Among the worst activities for low back cases are bending, sweeping, ironing, gardening, painting, polishing automobiles, and riding in most two-door cars on a seat that was designed to fold.

Gentle exercises as outlined later may be started 6 to 8 weeks after treatment. (See written post-treatment instructions in back of book.)

Discretion in Technic

With a knowledge of the anatomy and following the technic as outlined, there should not be any unfavorable result from injecting the proliferant solution within the ligaments and tendons.

(1) The solution is *distributed* at various points of attachment to bone, and there is no pooling of any considerable amount of the solution in one small area.

(2) Most of the proliferant injections are begun while the point of the needle is against bone. In some thick ligaments, injection is continued while withdrawing the point of the needle throughout the ligament. Tendon attachments are not thick, and the injection is made only while the point of the needle is in contact with bone.

There are no blood vessels or nerves of any size or importance within the ligament and tendon attachments to bone. Most relaxation occurs and the treatment is given dorsal to the bone, while the important nerves and blood vessels lie ventral to the bones.

(3) As in all therapy, there are a few areas in which unfavorable sequelae could result if the technic is not followed: (a) In the upper cervical area between the occiput and the third cervical vertebra, a needle missing the bone if directed deeply enough could contact important nerves and blood vessels. Most of the relaxation occurs below the third cervical where the lamina and transverse processes are in close proximity and slide over one another. (b) A needle inserted too deeply might penetrate the interspinus ligament and enter the spinal canal. (c) A needle missing the dorsal articular ligaments could contact a radicular nerve. Acute pain would warn the operator, and the needle would be redirected. (d) In the region of the fifth lumbar transverse process, a needle missing bone could contact important nerves which would elicit shooting pain into the foot, or if in a blood vessel, it would be noted on aspiration. One should have a mental picture of depth in each individual and each location. (e) The sacral foramen are rarely entered because the needle is usually directed at an angle. If in doubt, redirect the needle. (f) Injecting the posterior sacroiliac ligament (Fig. 1-D) on the outer side of the ilium above and medial to the sciatic foramen is only made when the needle is against bone to avoid contacting the sciatic nerve and blood vessels.

Additional Observation on Referred Pain

The illustrations and discussion on referred pain areas and sciatic pain from relaxation of specific articular ligaments of the lumbar spine and pelvis which were presented earlier in this edition was limited to those areas which I have found to occur most frequently, to be most representative, and to be most useful in diagnosis by directing attention to the source of pain.

There were other observations and impressions that were not included because they occur less often, their origin is variable or not definitely established, and their inclusion might have contributed more confusion than assistance to the reader.

Some confusion in determining the precise origin of certain referred pains lies in the fact that the strands of adjoining ligaments are interlaced. Also the point of the needle may reach them from different insertions. These areas are: the upper sacroiliac notch; the notch between the posterior superior spine of the ilium and the sacrum; at the lower margin of the sacroiliac joint; and the close relationship of the piriformis muscle and its tendon attachments with the sciatic nerve, the ligaments at the lower portion of the sacroiliac joint, and the articular ligament of the hip joint.

The variations may have their origin in the innervation of ligament strands that are less frequently relaxed, or perhaps in variations of innervation or susceptibility of nerve stimulation from other spinal segments.

I will present some of the observations so that when the reader encounters them he will have a better understanding of the related variations which I have observed to occur less frequently. They may also be helpful to future investigators to improve the dermatomes as we now understand them.

Critics should know and future investigators may be interested in knowing that it has required thousands of observations, while diagnosing and treating hundreds of patients, to acquire the data to make possible the construction of these dermatomes. And during that time, we have been engaged in recording observations on different proliferants and anesthetics, and in improving our diagnostic acumen and technic of treatment.

In addition there were scientific presentations, instructing visiting physicians, animal experimentation, and a voluminous correspondence.

An increase of staff might have enabled us to train more doctors and treat more patients, but it was concluded that it might also interrupt our observations which it seemed necessary to continue. Consequently, these presentations are the product of one individual with the invaluable assistance of one nurse-secretary.

Our observations on referred pain from the relaxed articular ligaments of the cervical and dorsal spine and the related skeletal tendons has revealed them to extend upward into the head and outward into the upper extremities including the fingers, and into the chest and abdomen and their anterior walls.

Referred pain from the occipital and upper cervical ligaments and tendons is referred into the head including eye pain (Fig. 25). The middle and lower cervical ligaments have referred pain into specific areas of the upper extremity. Knowledge of the referred pain areas from the cervical and dorsal skeleton have been less useful in diagnosis by directing attention to the origin of pain in specific ligaments and tendons, such as is so valuable in low back disability. For diagnosis in this area the trigger point tenderness is most important, and it is more easily obtained than in the low back because it is more superficial.

It is very important, however, to know that the cause of the disability has been identified, when we reproduce the local and referred pain by needling, for it is convincing and warrants the proper treatment.

The important thing to realize is that so much disability of the neck and back is due to ligament and tendon relaxation that it must be considered in the evaluation of any back pain. And for emphasis, I will state that no one can possibly realize how much pain between the skull and the coccyx is due to relaxation of the attachment of soft tissue to the bone until he has become competently able to diagnose it.

It has been recognized that there is a relationship between visceral stimulation and cutaneous hyperalgesia since the work of my mentor, Sir Henry Head, and Sir James Mackenzie. It had not been recognized that somatic pain from *ligament relaxation* was referred to viscera and affected the normal function. I have found gastric distress that was reproduced by needling the 6th dorsal interspinus ligament.

The most frequent disturbance of visceral function that I have encountered occurs in the lower colon as a result of referred pain that has its origin in afferent sensory branches of the 12th dorsal nerve which are located in the ilial attachment of the ilio-lumbar ligament. Less often the origin is in the interspinus ligament of the 12th dorsal and 1st lumbar vertebrae. The most frequent bowel manifestation is an uncomfortable sensation or distress in the low abdomen accompanied by gas. There is frequently an accompanying constipation. The pain in the intestine and testicle have been reproduced by needling in the dorsal 12th, lumbar articular and the iliolumbar ligaments, and the tendon attachments to the transverse processes of all the lumbar vertebrae, and the constipation and testicle pain have entirely cleared up on treatment. My attention was first directed to it by a physician and his wife, who were both treated at the same time for similar lumbosacral instability involving the iliolumbar ligament (Cases #25 and #26). Another patient with involvement of the 12th dorsal interspinus ligament described the discomfort as a lump in the abdomen on either side just below the umbilicus.

Cardiac embarrassment can result from somatic pain stimulation in the 4th dorsal interspinus ligament.

Referred pain from the iliolumbar ligament commonly manifests itself as discomfort in the testicle in the male and one side of the vagina in the female. It may also occasionally result in a pain in the penis or a tugging (pulling down) sensation at the base of the penis accompanying the testicle pain. The ovary receives its innervation from the 10th dorsal segment and is not involved in iliolumbar ligament relaxation.

There is a definite relation between lumbosacral relaxation and bladder pain with frequent urge to void but is unrelieved on voiding. It has been reproduced on needling and cleared up entirely 12 days after treatment.

One vaginal pain was worse during the menstrual period for 29 years. She could only kneel in church by pressing the buttock against the seat, which rotated the lower sacrum forward and the upper sacrum backward which relieved the strain on the iliolumbar ligament from which the vaginal referred pain had its origin. Sometimes the groin pain seems to push down into the side of the vagina, and the vagina pain has felt like a pushing out through the orifice but is most often a burning or numbness. The low abdomen pain from the iliolumbar ligament may result in nausea if the inducing strain is continued. The testicle discomfort may be numb, tickling, itching, burning, pulling, or aching.

Rectal pain may be associated with lumbosacral ligament relaxation, but more often with relaxation of the lower sacral ligaments.

Pain on the inside of the knee, most often over the upper end of the tibia, is associated with lumbosacral relaxation, the upper sacroiliac relaxation, and relaxation of the adductor longus tendon at the descending ramus of the pubes. Once it was reproduced from the upper sacroiliac notch as being the size of a silver dollar on the inside and a dime on the outside but not running through the knee like a nail as sometimes occurs in cases of sciatica. The medial pain occurs more often and is always larger than the outer pain.

The sacroiliac relaxation, particularly at its lower margin, may have a transmitted pain into the lower abdomen accompanied by tenderness. There is a similar pain and tenderness *beneath* Poupart's ligament in the outer groin from hip disability. It should not be confused with the groin pain referred from the iliolumbar ligament which is higher and medial, just above Poupart's ligament.

I do not know of any referred pain back of the knee. It is always sciatic in the popliteal space and is usually more tender than in the thigh. I consider it a sciatic trigger point medially and laterally, and it accounts for various pains distal to the calf which do not fit diagnostically into any pattern, such as those on either side of the Achilles Tendon.

I have not found any referred pain of diagnostic value from the ligaments in the area of the posterior superior spine, although they appear in the rectum and perineum and can be reproduced on needling.

Usually when one of the central toes is more painful than the others in referred pain, it is because there is an accompanying tenderness of the associated metatarsal from a relaxed arch or callous, and the pain threshold has been lowered by long over-stimulation.

A left testicle had been degenerated to one-fourth the size of the right following an orchitis secondary to mumps 25 years previously. It was more highly sensitive on palpation than the right. There was much more referred pain in the left testicle than the right from relaxation of the iliolumbar ligaments, although the ligament and tendon local pain, referred pain and sciatica were more severe on the right side.

Severe referred pain in the left testicle was reproduced by needling the left articular ligaments and transverse process tendons from the 12th dorsal vertebra to the 5th lumbar vertebra, while similar needling on the more sensitive right side did not reproduce pain in the right testicle.

From many similar observations I have concluded that abnormal prolonged overstimulation of the sensory nerve receptors of body tissue heightens not only its susceptibility to additional painful stimuli, but also heightens the susceptibility of its anterior horn ganglion to receive extraneous impulses from other nerves entering the same ganglion which are transmitted to the brain and interpreted as referred pain.

Sometimes patients who have abdominal disorders that are considered independent of their lumbar somatic disability report that the abdominal disturbance has abated after the lumbar ligament and tendon relaxation has been eliminated by Prolotherapy.

It is well known that some patients have observed headaches to be associated with bowel disturbances. We now know of the association of bowel disturbances with lumbar and lumbosacral somatic disability. In some cases the patients report that the headaches as well as the abdominal discomfort have abated following lumbar Prolotherapy. A sufficient number of cases have not been followed long enough to arrive at definite conclusions, but the correlation deserves further study.

On re-examination, evidence of benefit from treatment is found in the absence, diminution of intensity or frequency of referred pain such as is found in the eyes, scalp, headaches, dizziness, fingers and upper extremity, testicle, vagina, bladder, abdominal discomfort, groin, toes, feet or anywhere in the lower extremity. It is also an excellent check on the patient who does not realize he has improved but has confined his thinking to any remaining discomfort which sometimes has not been treated. Complete records should be kept. Severe and/or long standing sciatica (conducted pain) may persist for a considerable length of time, even after the referred and local pains have noticeably diminished. Patience along with additional treatment, together with avoidance of aggravating activities, will be rewarding.

Animal Experiments

To explain the modus operandi and clinical results that had been obtained over a period of 13 years by the injection of a proliferating solution within the posterior ligaments of the lumbar and sacral articulations, a series of animal experiments were begun in 1952.

There was a need for this investigation because, although both the patients and I were satisfied that the clinical results of proliferation of ligaments in the stabilization of relaxed joints was entirely satisfactory, it became increasingly evident that some physicians were skeptical of the method.

It, therefore, seemed advisable to present evidence of the manner in which the clinical results were accomplished.

Also no previous scientific work had been done which demonstrated the volume of strong fibrous tissue which could be generated by the introduction of a proliferant within the articular ligaments, although the experiments had been made on other tissue which revealed the production of strong fibrous tissue.

The experimental work has been carried out on tendons because there are no ligaments in the smaller animals which are of sufficient size and accessability to carry out the experiments. Ligaments and tendons are composed of nonelastic white fibrous tissue, both are attached to bones, and both become similarly disabled.

The rabbit was selected for the investigation, and the experiments were made on the gastrocnemius and superficial flexor tendons where they are conjoined to the tuber calcanei of the tibial tarsal bone, analogous to the Achilles Tendon in man. The technic was similar to that used clinically in which both the local anesthetic and the proliferating solution were injected within the fibrous bundles of the tendon. The tissue work and photography were done by Henderson.

Microphotographs of sections represent the effect of proliferating action on the tissues in the formation of permanent bone and fibrous tissue.

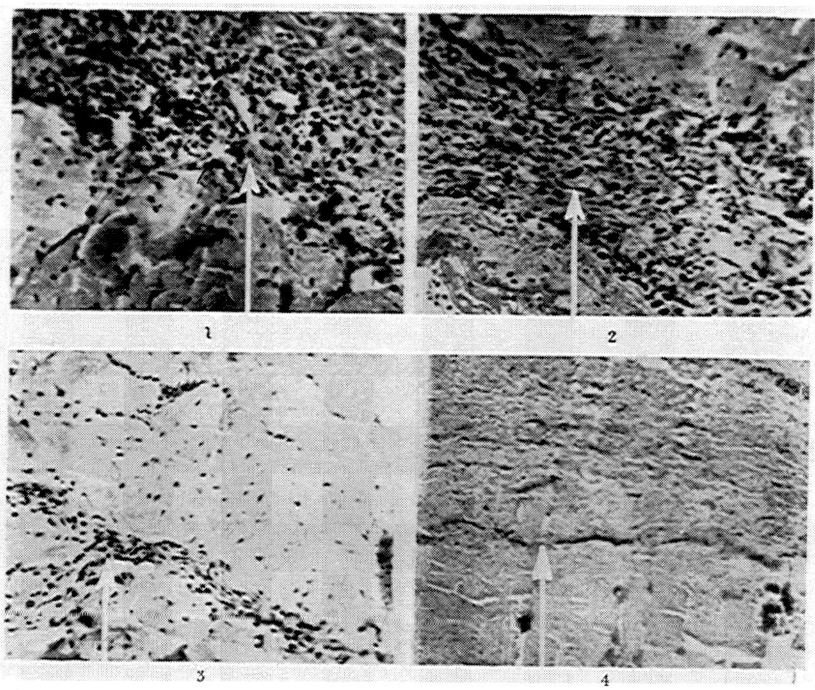

Fig. 29 (1-2-3-4). Microphotographs of sections from rabbit tendons following the injection of the proliferant, Sylnasol (G. D. Searle & Co.), within the fibrous strands. The same technic was used as that which is used clinically.

1) Arrow points to moderate infiltration of lymphocytes 48 hours after injection of proliferating solution. Note absence of necrosis in surrounding tissue.

2) Beginning fibroplastic organization present in adjacent tissues. Arrow points to capillary proliferation with moderate infiltration of lymphocytes. Two weeks after injection.

3) Fibrous tissue now present. Lymphocytic infiltration minimal. One month after injection. Arrow points to few fibroblasts.

4) Fibrosis now present, lymphocytes absent and sheath thickened and fibrosed nine months after initial injection. Arrow points to junction of tendon and its sheath. Nine months after initial injections.

Photographs and x-rays reveal the gross production of permanent bone and fibrous tissue.

In 1955 Hackett and Henderson reported two years animal experimentation on the effects of the proliferant, Sylnasol, when injected within the fibrous strands of rabbits tendons. They reported the absence of necrosis or destruction of nerves, blood vessels or tendonous bands. In 48 hours histological examination (Fig. 29, 1) revealed an early inflammatory reaction surrounding the nerves and blood vessels with lymphocytic infiltration throughout the area between the two tendons and between the tendon and its sheath.

Two weeks after the injection (Fig. 29, 2) fibrous tissue was present, lymphocytic infiltration had diminished although some was still present which indicated that the proliferation of new white fibrous tissue was still being stimulated.

One month after injection, (Fig. 29, 3) fibrous tissue was present; lymphocytic and fibroplastic activity was greatly diminished.

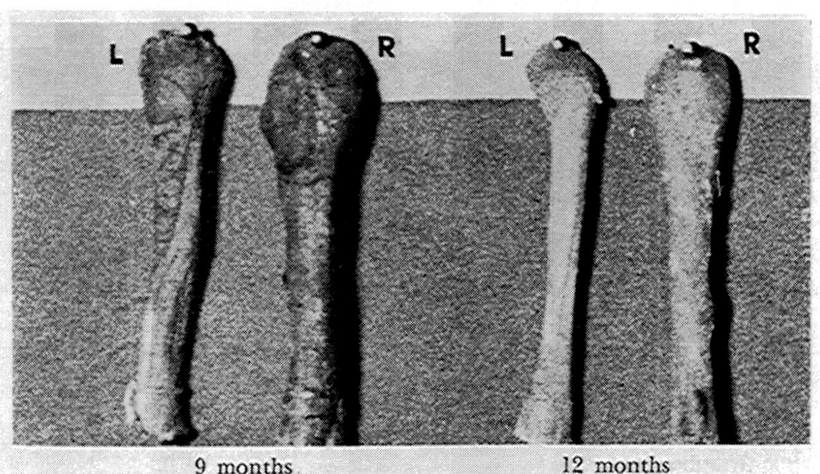

Fig. 30. Photograph of rabbit tendons at nine and 12 months after three injections of proliferating solution into the right tendons. *Left,* controls; *right,* proliferated. The tendons on the right reveal an increase in diameter of 40 per cent, which is estimated to double the strength of the tendon. The upper portion reveals the attachment of the ligament to the bone which has increased 30 per cent in diameter. The proliferating solution stimulates the production of new fibrous connective tissue cells which become organized into permanent non-elastic fibrous tissue.

Sections at nine months (Fig. 29, 4) revealed permanent white fibrous tissue had formed, and there was no inflammatory process present.

Quantitatively, the results at the end of nine and 12 months (Fig. 30) as compared with controls in the same rabbit which were not injected revealed an increase of 40 per cent in diameter of the tendons which were injected with the proliferating solution.

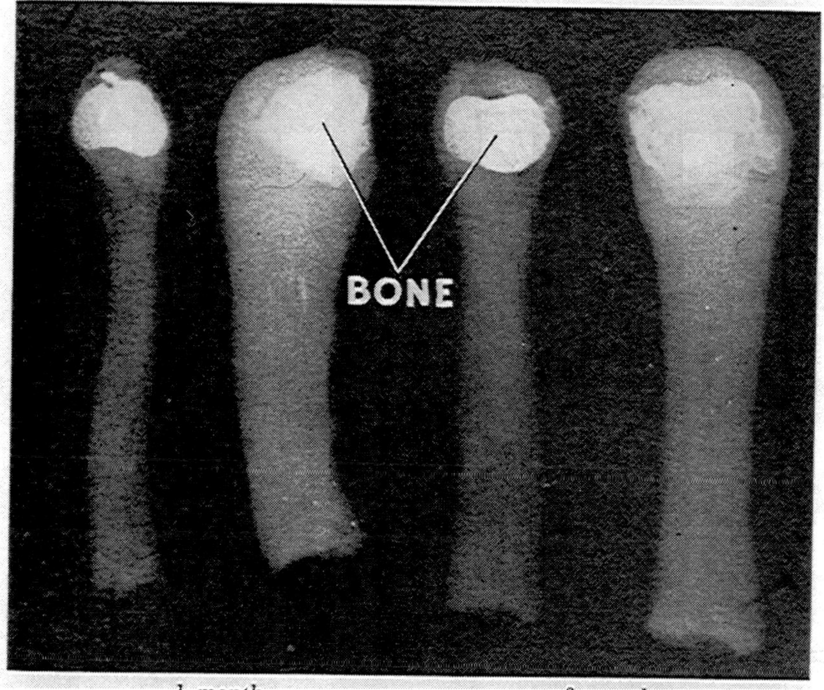

Fig. 31. Roentgenograms of the proximal end of the tibial tarsal bone of the rabbit with the attached gastrocnemius and superficial flexor tendons. The films were made one and three months after a single injection of proliferant solution had been distributed throughout the tendon.

They reveal a marked increase of bone at one month as compared with the control and a further increase of bone at three months.

The increase in soft tissue at one month was pronounced due to the presence of new fibrous tissue cells, while at three months the increase is due to the production of permanent fibrous tissue.

The increase of bone was significant because it resulted in a strong fibro-osseous union ("weld") where sprains, tears and relaxation of the ligament chiefly take place and where the sensory nerves are abundant.

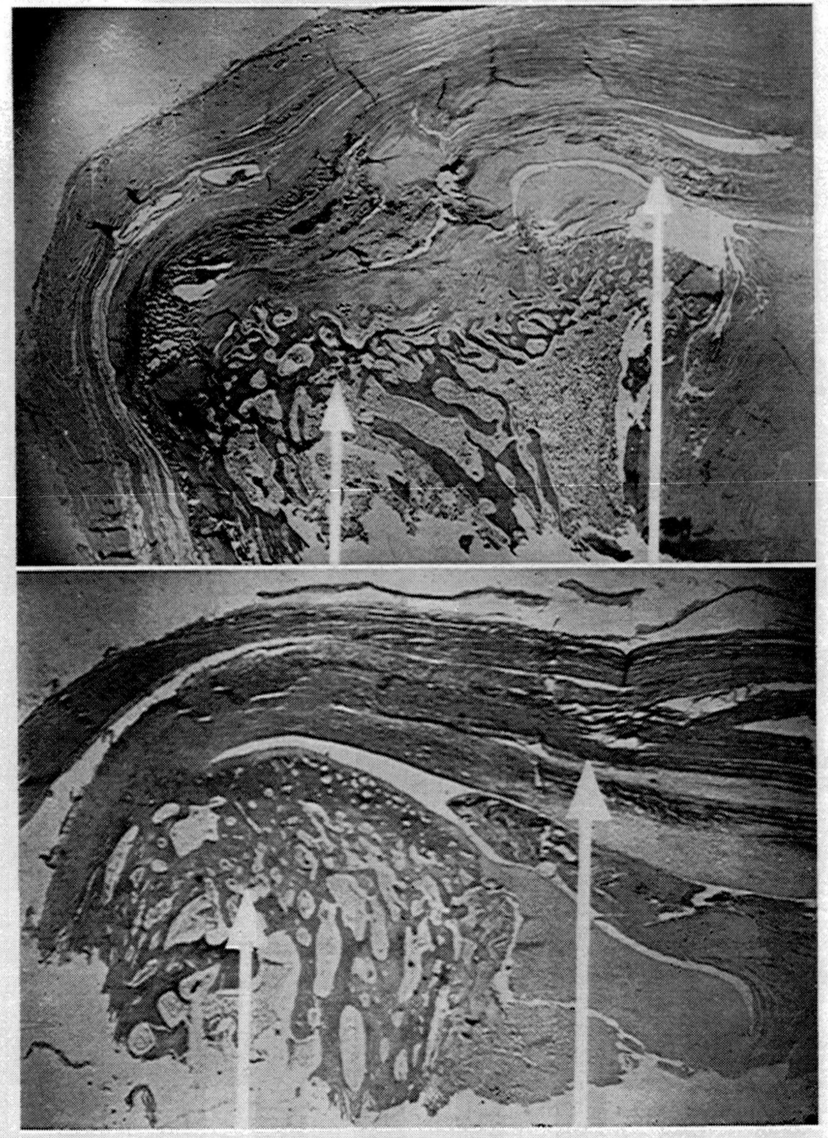

Fig. 32. *Animal Experimentation.*

Two microphotographs of the gastrocnemius and superficial flexor tendons attached to the tibial tarsal bones of a rabbit two months after one of
them had been injected with a proliferant solution.

Following decalcification, the sections were made from the central part of
the end of the bone together with its tendon attachment, the fibro-osseous
junction.

Below is a decalcified tissue section from the *control* leg. The end of the
bone is shown on the left (short arrow).

One the right is shown the fibrous tissue (long arrow) as it swings over and around the bone to its anterior surface on the left where the attachment is made to the bone.

The fibers of the tendon are continuous through the periosteum with the fibrous matrix of the bone (Cunningham's Anatomy).

Above is a decalcified tissue section from the leg which received one injection of the proliferant solution (Sylnasol, G. D. Searle & Co.). The same technic was followed as is used clinically.

The injection was made from above and was distributed down through the fibrous tissue and along the posterior edge of the bone, through the area shown by the long arrow.

The proliferant stimulated the production of new bone and fibrous tissue cells at the fibro-osseous junction which became permanent.

At two months it reveals an abundant increase of the fibrous connection between the tendon and the fibrous bone matrix. This gives a stronger "weld" at the fibro-osseous junction and accounts for the clinical results obtained.

In the end of the tendon with its attachment to bone, the increase in diameter was 30 per cent.

Also included in the article was a report and a photostat of x-rays of rabbit tendons (Fig. 31) which were taken at periods of one and three months after injection of the proliferating solution at the fibro-osseous junction, as compared with controls in the same rabbit which were not injected.

The x-rays revealed a marked increase of bone as well as fibrous tissue at both one and three months. At the end of three months the inflammatory reaction was absent.

A microphotograph (Fig. 32) of decalcified bone and tendon shows sections from the proliferated tissue and control at two months. There is revealed a marked increase of both bone and fibrous tissue in the proliferated section as compared with the control.

Of particular significance is the great increase of continuous fibrous tissue which extends from the tendon, through the periosteum, into the bone to increase the strength of the "weld."

The proliferation of bone and fibrous tissue taking place at the same time while overlapping or invading each other at their point of junction would produce a "weld" of the two tissues which would increase the strength significantly at its weakest point.

The results of these experiments were demonstrated in booths of the scientific sections at the Ohio State Medical Convention in 1955 in Cincinnati; at the annual meetings of The American Medical Association in Atlantic City in 1955 and in New York in 1957; at the American Academy of General Practice meetings in Washington, D.C. in 1956 and in St. Louis in 1957; at the clinical session of the American Medical Association in Boston in 1955; at the Interstate Postgraduate Medical Association in Milwaukee in 1955, and at the Southern Medical Association Meeting in Miami Beach in 1957. It has also been presented at the scientific sessions of the annual meetings of The American Medical Association in 1955, at The New Brunswick (Canada) Annual Meeting in 1956, at the International College of Surgeons meeting in 1956, and at the American College of Surgeons meeting in Toledo in 1957.

History of Proliferation

The therapeutic production of fibrous tissue by the injection of a stimulating solution was begun in 1832 by Jaynes of St. Louis, who used essential oils and later a tincture in the injection treatment of hernia before the days of asepsis, which was accepted by 1890, and of general anesthesia which together made possible the successful operative treatment of hernia.

In the early days the name "sclerosing solution" was given to any solution which produced abundant fibrous tissue because it resembled scar tissue formation, and the aim in treatment was to produce a strong tissue which would withstand pressure and prevent a bulging at the external inguinal ring. The sclerosing treatment was applied to a variety of disabilities with varying success. It is still successfully used in the treatment of varicose veins.

The action of the stimulating solution has always been that of a proliferant, which Webster's *Dictionary* defines biologically as the production of new cells in rapid succession.

I prefer to designate the action on ligaments and bone as one of proliferation because it describes the therapeutic action which is desired and obtained in strengthening the fibrous tissue and bone at the fibro-osseous junction and to which I applied the name *prolotherapy* in 1956.

It appears that Velpeau of France in 1835 was given credit as the originator of the injection treatment of hernia before the work of Jaynes was published.

A scientific rationale for the use of a proliferant was established in 1881 when Warren reported the study of tissue reaction to the injection of "Quercus Alba." This reaction was characterized by the early formation of "plastolymph"; this later became organized into fibrous tissue which acquired strength in 10 to 12 days.

Mayer in 1900 used a zinc sulfate, phenol solution in the injection treatment of hernia with considerable success in selected cases.

In 1929 Hall and Frazier using guinea pigs, monkeys and dogs demonstrated the vigorous proliferation of endothelial and connective tissue cells following the injection of a proliferating solution. These experiments were verified and elaborated in 1936 by Harris and White and in 1938 by Harris, White and Biskind and by Maniol and by others who compared the histological and side effects of different proliferating solutions. Harris and his associates showed that the main mass of proliferating fibrous tissue was located in the connective tissue septa.

Rice in 1935 investigated human tendons and fascia and observed the progressive effects of various solutions on the tissues at periods ranging from 15 hours to 42 days. He observed that the tissue reaction induced by proliferants follows the laws of inflammation. The reaction of connective tissue cells is one of permanence and contractility. This investigation revealed, along with the others previously mentioned, that the ideal solution was one that had the following desirable features: (1) causes a minimum of early exudate, (2) a minimum of discomfort, (3) stimulates a maximum of permanent white fibrous connective tissue, (4) no systemic reaction, and (5) no sloughing or destruction of tissue.

In 1939 when I came to the conclusion that some low back disability was due to relaxation of the posterior sacroiliac ligaments, I initiated the method of strengthening the ligaments by the intraligamentous injection of a proliferating solution. Within a short time the method showed evidence of being successful. The disabilities of the patients were relieved; they were able to resume their previous activities which had been necessarily restricted. They continued to remain free of disability until they had no more recurrence and were pronounced cured. The treatment was extended to include ligaments of all the articulations of the spine and pelvis and many other joints of the skeleton.

In 1955 I came to the conclusion that the tendons of muscles become relaxed at their attachment to bone similarly to ligaments, and since that time we have been successful in strengthening them by Prolotherapy in various locations of the skeleton.

I have been unable to conduct a satisfactory survey since the one made four years ago, but with the improvement in diagnosis and technic it is my considered judgment that we are now obtaining cures that are entirely satisfactory to the patients in over 90 per cent of the cases treated. Rarely are the patients dissatisfied, and only a few fail to complete the course of treatment until satisfaction has been attained.

History of Ligament Treatment

The treatment of joint instability (ligament relaxation) for ages in the past has been bandaging, splints, braces, casts and adhesive plaster to restrict motion and support the joint. Also liniment, heat, massage and physiotherapy have been used. Exercises have been used in an attempt to strengthen the ligaments with little success for the strain is more likely to induce pain and increase the weakness, so that exercises are rarely continued.

With the advent of anesthesia in the past century, some operations have been devised on plicating ligaments, but the operations are chiefly of the fusion type and have had the effect of weakening the ligamentous support in the guise of strengthening the articulation.

Traction probably does not accomplish anything that cannot be obtained by rest in bed with analgesics and with greater comfort in a shorter period of time.

No spinal fusion operation in the past has survived its originator, nor will probably any now in vogue, nor any in the future, for most fusion operations impair function and usually result in limited activity and continued discomfort.

Eighteen years ago I decided that much of the low back pain and disability was due to relaxation of the articular ligaments and considered methods of strengthening them. Having had some experience in operating on cases of hernia which had previously been injected with a proliferating solution, I was impressed with the increased density and strength of the tissues which were encountered.

I applied the proliferating injection treatment to the relaxed ligaments by injecting the solution within the fibrous bands, and within a short time I was impressed with the clinical results obtained and the patients were most enthusiastic. I have improved the technic and extended the treatment to the posterior ligaments of all the joints of the spine and pelvis and several other joints with gratifying results.

The patients have usually been able to resume any previous activities which had been restricted or accompanied by pain.

When the ligaments become strengthened and the joint stabilized, there is rarely a recurrence unless the patient suffers an accident.

There is a dearth of information about the disability of ligaments in medical schools, postgraduate training and in medical literature including text books. Ligament disability, other than strains, is rarely mentioned. If the ligaments do not regain their normal stabilizing strength, the disability is referred to as a weak joint rather than weak ligaments. Efforts to permanently stabilize the articulation have been directed toward surgery, usually at the sacrifice of more ligament tissue or the bony processes to which the ligaments are attached for leverage, or both.

Schultz injected a proliferant into the temporomandibular joint cavity and produced a fibrogenesis in all the tissues, but there is no previous report of the stabilization of joints by injection within the ligaments of a proliferant which stimulated bone and fibrous tissue.

Résumé of Low Back Treatment

To properly understand the present situation it is advisable to review the history of low back treatment during the past half century as found in the literature and from personal observation during the past 40 years.

Fifty years ago belts, braces, elastics, heel lifts, adhesive plaster and plaster of Paris were used much as they are today. Following acceptance of antisepsis and the development of general anesthesia about 65 years ago, various bone fusion operations of the lumbosacral and sacroiliac joints were contrived and were in vogue with about the same results as are obtained today. Gaenslen in 1927 gave a test for sacroiliac disability which depended on relaxation of the ligaments and for which he described an arthrodesis which would preserve the posterior sacroiliac ligament. No other low back operation devised has shown such consideration for ligaments.

Eyes peering at the roentgenograms discovered the transverse process of the 5th lumbar vertebra to be fused with or lying close to the sacrum, and the pioneer surgeons removed them with abandon, as they do today, vertebral spines, portions of the articular processes, the top of sacrum with its attached ligaments and sometimes the discs. It was an effort to stabilize the spine and lumbosacral junction which resulted from relaxation of the ligaments as it does today according to Meisenbach.

Laminectomy operations were successfully performed for the removal of "condroma" (cartilaginous disc tumors) which pressed on the cord and radicular nerves, comparable to the operations of today.

Over two decades ago three ideas appeared which definitely changed the course of events in low back treatment. One was the description of the ruptured nucleus pulposus in 1934 as described by Mixter and Barr. It is a definite scientific entity and will endure. However, it has gotten out of control because of the confusion in diagnosis and has resulted in too many unsatisfactory operations. Barr pointed out in 1951 that, "Too many backs are being irretrievably damaged by ill-advised and ill-considered operations."

Another idea appeared a short time later and is mentioned only because of the confusion which resulted from it. It was an ethereal idea for which no scientific basis was even attempted. It was called "fibrositis," and to it was attributed all the many pain and disabilities which did not fall into the sphere of the ruptured disc, or to be explained by the vagaries of a roentgenogram. It was widely accepted and had a vocal band of followers who mushroomed it into a position of prominence which it could not maintain and so is withering away and rarely mentioned. Waters referred to it as a "catch-all term." Unfortunately most of those undiagnosed cases are now designated with such unscientific etherial terms as slipped, narrowed, crushed or possible ruptured discs, imaginary radicular nerve impingements, or visionary abnormalities as misinterpreted from the roentgenograms. They can be relegated to the waste basket along with "lumbago."

The third is an erroneous idea that crept in during the "fibrositic period" and took root with devastating consequences. It is the fallacy that very little disability can be accredited to the sacroiliac joint, when in reality more instability occurs in the sacroiliac joint than in the lumbosacral or any other articulation of the back. This was revealed by Steindler in 1925 when he reported three cases of sacroiliac disability to two cases of lumbosacral disability. My experience is comparable.

The cases with back disability will continue to gravitate to cults or endure their disabilities like they do today as long as this disorientation continues.

The mass production of unnecessary unsatisfactory spinal operations that were turned out in the post-war decade by the inexperienced surgeons, whose training was overemphasized on the mechanical side, helps to confuse the public and make them wary.

I am frequently consulted by patients who have had disc and spinal fusion operations by surgeons who do not consider the sacroiliac joint and its ligaments as causing any trouble.

These patients continue to have the same pain, referred pain and sciatica from relaxation of the ligaments that support the lumbosacral and sacroiliac articulations that they had previous to the operations.

I have successfully treated them in cases that have not been too extensively mutilated by operations which sacrifice important ligaments and bone prominences that have been developed to give leverage for attached ligaments and tendons.

The belief that the pain and disability of lumbosacral instability from ligament relaxation can be eliminated by lumbosacral fusion is erroneous. Even if the 5th lumbar vertebra was solidly fused by operation to the sacrum, there would remain the forward rotation of the upper sacrum at the sacroiliac joint. This would continue to place tension on the relaxed fibers of the iliolumbar and upper portion of the posterior sacroiliac ligaments, and frequently to a greater degree than before the fusion was performed. I have observed this in many patients including surgeons. The interspinus ligament pain may have been eliminated by excision.

If fusion operations for lumbosacral disability were to be successful, it would also be necessary to immobilize the sacroiliac joints at the same time. This was recognized in the aggressive sacral stabilization period of the first three decades of this century by Chandler in 1929 when he devised the trisacral fusion operation. This unsuccessful procedure has not yet been revived by the later entrepreneurs.

Reappeared is the medieval practice of "placing the victim on the rack" with traction. Its chief advantage is enforced rest in the prone position if it can be called rest. By periodically removing the traction the patient is able to relax and recover unless he has been driven by this deviltry to submit to a laminectomy or arthrodesis or both according to the vogue of his environment. Eminent orthopedic surgeons have informed me that they only use traction to get enforced rest. Spine operations may run to six depending on the credulity of the patients and the eagerness of the operator.

Ligaments which interfere with exposure are sacrificed. Spines, lamina, discs, and portions of the articular fulcrum of the vertebrae are laid waste with abandon. The tendons of muscles are incised or torn by traction and dissection from their bony attachments. Normal disc tissue is removed and replaced by artificial plastics or pounded full of bone chips. The ligament stabilization of the joint is destroyed under the pretense of correcting it, although Mixter and Barr originally warned, "A ruptured disc is a weakened disc, and the strength of the spine should be preserved—." Operations are running ahead of intelligent diagnosis.

Promiscuous "pot shot" intramuscular injections of local anesthetics, cortisone, and other easy to give pharmaceutical concoctions are in full swing. The latest "easy way" does not even require a physical examination or diagnosis. It is the ultrasonic vibrator which is held in one hand and moved over the skin until the patient announces the offending area where the mystic wave can be concentrated.

Two observations by Ghormley were prophetic. In 1944 he said, "As the widespread interest in lesions of the intervertebral disc has drawn increased attention to the lumbosacral joint, the importance of the sacroiliac joint as a source of symptoms has waned, perhaps to a point where sacroiliac conditions be overlooked."

Again in 1951, Ghormley stated that since the syndrome of the intervertebral disc has been recognized perhaps the diagnosis of sacroiliac strain "should not have been *abandoned* for undoubtedly the sacroiliac joint does cause symptoms at times."

Armstrong pointed out in 1951 that wrong diagnosis was the most common cause for failure in low back operations, and Scuderi recently opined that "the hope that spinal fusion will cure backache with pain radiating to the legs is an illusion." Gardner revealed that ligamentous strain in the vertebral region can give subjective pain similar to that from a ruptured disc but without the objective signs of root damage.

Since ligament relaxation is the most common cause of low back disability and the diagnosis can be verified, the existing confusion of low back diagnosis and treatment can be cleared up.

Interest in ligament disability which has been stimulated by the diagnosis and treatment of ligament relaxation during the past 19 years will make it possible to confine disc operations to the few low back disabilities for which it is appropriate, and the operation may again command a position of respect among the profession and the general public. Fusion operations of the spine and pelvis will be necessary for extreme disc degeneration and marked vertebral displacement. Satisfactory stabilization of the articulations by fibro-osseous proliferation will obviate the necessity for most fusion operations.

Within the past year I have encountered cases that had submitted to unsuccessful cordotomy operations after they had run the gamut of laminectomy and fusion procedures. Apparently the cordotomy operation is an attempt to dissociate the conscious perception of pain from its somatic origin in the low back articular ligaments, which had remained throughout all the contrivances and to which was added the tendon relaxation pain that resulted from the operations. In one case there resulted from the cordotomy an additional unbearable burning pain on the opposite side of the body below the cervical cordotomy which was electrified by the weight of a bedsheet at night or a crumpled bill or piece of paper in the pocket of his loose trousers.

Because of his marked tenderness the diagnosis of his relaxed joint ligaments and relaxed lumbar tendons was only possible from the local and referred pain areas which he described to me. Treatment was possible only under intravenous anesthesia.

Two months after the initial treatment, examination revealed that stabilization of his lumbosacral and sacroiliac joints and lumbar tendons had definitely reduced his local pain and obliterated most of his referred pain. Also alleviated to a considerable extent was the burning pain throughout the one side, after the somatic ligament and tendon sensory stimuli had been reduced.

Another case resulted in a partial paralysis of the lower extremity on the operated side following her second cordotomy.

Obviously the post-operative spine cases that visit my office are chiefly the failures, although a few have had protruding discs successfully removed with the radicular pain completely relieved, while their remaining disability was due to the articular ligament relaxation which had been present before the radicular pain induced by the disc.

Likewise it is only my failures that later are seen by others. There are a few cases in which I have stabilized the articulations and did not realize that a protruded disc was also present. These cases have the advantage that following their laminectomy operations their recovery should be complete because the joints have already been stabilized by prolotherapy. Some of these borderline cases may be troublesome until improved diagnosis can distinguish between them, because the "sciatica" accompanying relaxation of the ligaments that stabilize the lower portion of the sacroiliac joint is very similar to the radicular pain of the protruding disc. This accounts for many failures following exploratory laminectomy operations.

I had been referring doubtful disc cases to a competent neurosurgeon. Some of these cases had returned without operation, and I was able to cure them to their satisfaction by strengthening the ligaments.

This review of the situation as I have seen it has been given with the idea of "taking stock" so that with a better understanding we will be able to improve the diagnosis and treatment of low back disability. In doing so, I hope I have not tramped on too many tender toes.

Much thinking should be revised, as well as textbooks, to include the somatic disability of ligament and tendon relaxation at their bony attachments. By cooperation of teaching centers along with the medical journals and specialty sections that deal with skeletal disability, the medical profession would readily comprehend and adopt this basic medical concept.

Those cooperative journals included in the index as well as the scientific sections of medical associations where our presentations have been so enthusiastically received are to be commended.

Additional Considerations—Comment

Some of the following statements may be a recapitulation. They are added for emphasis.

The elimination of obesity with its additional weight and change of posture will eliminate a considerable amount of strain on various ligaments especially in the low back.

In severe cases with excessive pain and muscular spasticity, the diagnosis sometimes cannot be made until the acute symptoms have been controlled.

When accompanied by painful confining injuries, the symptoms of ligament relaxation may not appear until activities are begun, as when accompanying a severe fracture. Then they are usually attributed to the other injuries. As special examiner for approximately 70 accident insurance companies for over 30 years, I found that only a small per cent of the disabilities to the ligaments of the low back had been recognized.

When the point of the needle contacts bone, some of the proliferant is injected before the course of the needle is changed.

When a needle encounters an area in a ligament which had been injected previously, there is great resistance due to the firm fibrous tissue which has been proliferated.

The patients realize they have been cured and resume previously curtailed activities without discomfort. They report that they are free from symptoms and treatments are discontinued.

This is the first time in history that articular ligaments and tendons have been successfully strengthened. It is also the initial success in bone proliferation.

In back diagnosis, much has been known about muscles, bones, discs, the spinal cord and fluid, and the nerves emanating from the cord. To learn about the ligaments is like fitting the final word in a crossword puzzle. All becomes clear. But, without this knowledge, the diagnosis of back disability will continue in confusion, and the treatment, whether medical or surgical, will continue to be unsatisfactory in too many cases.

As previously stated under Diagnosis and Treatment, lumbosacral and upper sacroiliac joint instability occur so frequently together that one must always consider when dealing with one whether the other is also involved.

Severe sacroiliac instability can occur alone, but severe lumbosacral instability rarely occurs without an accompanying instability of the upper portion of the sacroiliac joint on one or both sides. Also severe relaxation of the lumbosacral and sacroiliac ligaments may be present together on one side, while on the other side there may not be any relaxation of the sacroiliac ligaments and slight if any relaxation of the iliolumbar and lumbosacral ligaments.

There is a normal synchronizing forward movement of the upper portion of the sacrum away from the ilium at the same time the 5th lumbar vertebra glides forward at its articulation with the sacrum. This synchronized movement is under the stabilizing control of the interlacing ligaments of the three bones: the ilium, the sacrum, and the 5th lumbar vertebra. There are ligaments from each bone that connect it with each of the other bones. These ligaments practically fill the deep space beneath the sacrospinus muscle known as the iliolumbar triangle. They have their attachments to the posterior and lateral surface of the body of the 5th lumbar vertebra, its spine, transverse and articular processes, the top and posterior surface of the sacrum as well as the upper grooved area of the sacrum that forms the notch with the ilium above the sacroiliac joint, together with the ilium on its anterior surface beneath the crest which includes the area that helps to form the notch with the sacrum above the sacroiliac joint.

In this large notch between the sacrum and ilium above the sacroiliac joint, ligaments from all three bones are joined and cooperate in support of the synchronizing movement of flexion and rotation of both the lumbosacral and sacroiliac joints.

There may be some conflicting interpretation of the referred pain from this notch area, because the needle enters it both from above medially when inserted into the iliolumbar ligament (Fig. 1-IL-4), and from below medially when inserting it into the upper and outer fibers of the posterior sacroiliac ligament (Fig. 1-SI-High-1).

Most whiplash injuries of the neck which do not recover within three months are due to ligament and tendon relaxation. Many shoulder and upper arm disabilities that are considered to be bursitis are due to ligament or tendon relaxation and respond to proliferative treatment.

It should be mentioned that intercourse is one of the normal functions that is impaired in low back ligament disability and is restored following joint stabilization.

In back disability cases where a protrusion of a disc is questionable but relaxation of ligaments is obvious, the ligaments should first be strengthened by prolotherapy. In obvious cases of disc protrusion, a laminectomy should be done immediately.

Cases with active bone inflammation at the articulation accompanying ligament relaxation should have their ligaments strengthened to relieve the abnormal pressure, in such cases as slight disc narrowing. The articulation should be adequately supported by a brace, and activities should be limited during the prolonged period while the bone inflammation is subsiding. The results of strengthening ligaments in the presence of marked disc and bone degeneration are disappointing. These cases may respond favorably to spinal fusion.

Some critics of prolotherapy, in which new bone and fibrous tissue cells are being successfully stimulated, are themselves depending on what they call scar tissue formation (without new bone stimulation) to accomplish post-operative strength following spinal fusion operations.

Ligament and tendon relaxation and its treatment can be controversial only in minds that do not comprehend it.

May I suggest that prolotherapy be given a trial in delayed union and as an additional stimulant to the formation of new bone accompanying operations for non-union. I am unable to do this, for I am no longer engaged in skeletal operative surgery.

A young lady with an unstable knee joint causing total disability for 2 years was provided a rigid knee brace at a renowned clinic. Examination revealed relaxed anterior crucial and collateral ligaments which are being treated by Prolotherapy. After 8 months, re-evaluation reveals improved stabilization of the joint with less pain and more activity

Trigger point tenderness was located at the patellar ligament attachments to the lower margins of the patella bilaterally and the upper margins of the tibia tubercle bilaterally together with the medial and lateral expansion of the quadratus tendon attachments to the tibia.

The diagnosis was confirmed by needling, and proliferation treatment was given. She is now convalescing. This is the first knee treated by fibro-osseous proliferation. We anticipate a favorable outcome.

Trigger point pain or referred pain from ligaments which exists six weeks after treatment indicates additional treatment is needed.

Some patients state that as a result of the injection there is a numbness in the area several weeks later. It took me 17 years to determine that what once was a severe pain from the ligament before treatment was later perceived as a numbness when the ligament was only partly strengthened. Following another treatment the numbness also disappears.

Among the undiagnosed cases of ligament disability that I encounter, some have become drug addicts; others have been advised to consult psychiatrists, or seek sex gratification for supposed frustration. Others have been prescribed impossible exercises with accompanying generalized illustrations that only aggravate their painful ligaments, or are told that nothing can be done except to learn to live with it and to return for an operation if it got worse.

They come in with sacroiliac braces when they have only lumbosacral instability, and rigid spine braces when the disability is confined to one sacroiliac articulation.

Men with pain in the testicle from a relaxed iliolumbar ligament have been submitted to prostatic massage, cystoscopic, and kidney examinations, while the women with referred pain in the vagina have been submitted to cervical treatment, currettments and gynecological abdominal operations without relief.

Fully half the patients with low back ligament disability have either had spine operations performed or recommended, or have been advised that they had a ruptured, "slipped" or "crushed" disc.

"Slipped disc" is not a diagnosis but a convenient term to use when the cause of the pain and disability is not understood. It is in the same category as lumbago and syndromes (as currently used).

During the past two years my observations have been especially directed toward coordinating the referred pain areas and the areas of conducted sciatic pain from ligament and tendon disabilities. The considerable amount of data that was accumulated during the past year from 522 new cases along with that from cases in the previous year has enabled me to construct the dermatomes (Figs. 2 to 11) and trigger points (Fig. 1, 25, 26) which are presented in this edition. I believe they will permanently endure, and each year will be used to a greater extent in diagnosis as they become appreciated.

The physican who understands ligament and tendon disability and the associated referred pain and sciatica, as well as the associated anatomical components, will be able to diagnose back disability with confidence.

Sacrospinalis muscle—tendon—nerves. Probably no muscle and its tendon attachments to the skeleton has been so ignomineously dealt with by surgeons as the sacrospinalis when it has been surreptitiously removed from the dorsal surface of the sacrum and the spines and transverse processes of the vertebrae by bluntly severing its tendon attachments and nerves to approach a suspected obnoxious disc or an unstable joint whose causative factor was not understood. After defacing the skeleton, no adequate repair of the severed tendons, nerves and ligaments has been possible, or attempted. They are abandoned to their own misery. How much better to apply a less devastating therapy!

I am fully convinced that our present knowledge of ligaments and tendons will result in a reduction of spine operations by 90 per cent, similar to that of goiter and mastoid surgery. Resistance by patients has already reduced unnecessary, unsuccessful spinal fusion operations approximately 50 per cent. Every orthopedic surgeon who has visited us to be treated and/or observed our work has enthusiastically adopted the method. In addition to successfully using it, Compere had advised it editorially.

The dilemma of the orthopedic operative approach to spinal instability is presented on page 210 of the October 1957 issue of the *Cleveland Clinic Quarterly* which states that "Since Hibbs first proposed spinal fusion in 1911, the problems inherent in the operation have heretofore remained essentially unsolved".

Cortisone preparations allay inflammatory pain in acute conditions but should not be used in the treatment of chronic ligament and tendon relaxation because it retards and diminishes the normal process of fibro-osteogenetic proliferation which can be stimulated only by prolotherapy. This has been demonstrated in our present series of animal studies in Mercy Hospital.

The use of Cortisone in acute sprains should be avoided because it interferes with the normal repair of tissues.

Statistics

Ages range from 15 to 88 years. The third, fourth, fifth and sixth decades predominate.

Women comprise slightly more cases than men.

The average duration of disability was 4½ years. The longest period was 65 years; the shortest being 3 months.

Eighty-two per cent of the patients considered themselves cured over a period up to 12 years. The survey was made at the end of 14 years so that no cure was of less than 2 years' duration. Some of those cases have now remained cured for 19 years. No survey has been made recently, but we believe the number considering themselves cured is approximately 90 per cent due to our experience in diagnosis and improved technic of treatment.

A survey of 146 consecutive cases of undiagnosed low back disability over a 2-month period in 1955, with a distribution from the Atlantic to Pacific and Gulf States, revealed that 94 per cent had joint ligament relaxation. The average duration of disability was 10 years. One had submitted to four spine operations.

A survey of 137 consecutive cases of undiagnosed low back disability from the State of Michigan over a 4-month period in 1956 revealed that 97 per cent had joint instability from ligament relaxation. One had submitted to three spine operations.

In low back articular ligament relaxation, the sacroiliac joint instability is present in 75 per cent of the cases; lumbosacral joint instability in 54 per cent.

Approximately half of the patients with undiagnosed low back ligament disability have had a previous diagnosis of disc disability. Some have had as many as six spine operations, including laminectomy, arthrodesis, and cordotomy.

Sixteen hundred fifty six patients have been treated over a 19-year period. Approximately 18,000 intraligamentous injections have been made.

Failures can be attributed to (1) inability to clearly confirm the diagnosis by the injection of a local anesthetic solution, (2) failure of the patient to return for completion of the treatment, (3) treatment in the presence of another possible or known disability, (4) a less refined technic and less experience in the earlier studies, (5) years of suffering, combined with disappointments following treatment including operations, dependence on drugs, and abnormal living lead to a lowered morale, and (6) some individuals may not respond to the stimulation of proliferation, as do others.

Case Reports

Case 1. An executive, aged 51. The symptoms, of 20 years duration, had begun when he was carrying a piano. The pain was referred down the lateral aspect of the thigh and leg when he was carrying objects such as a heavy traveling bag. He alternately wore three sacroiliac belts. He had five injections in a period of three weeks, after which he was able to play golf without a sacroiliac belt. He remained cured for eight years and died of a cerebral accident.

Case 2. A nurse, aged 32. The symptoms, of eight months duration, had developed while she was lifting a heavy patient from floor to bed. Upon her admission to the hospital, two orthopedic surgeons diagnosed a disc injury and advised operation. An injection of novocaine with saline into the caudal canal resulted in no benefit. The patient had eight proliferating injections into the left sacroiliac ligaments within one month, during which time she was working. She was remained cured for eleven years. When she was last seen, in January 1957, she was engaged in her occupation as a nurse.

Case 3. A woman, aged 40, a taxicab driver, stopped suddenly for a red light, and her cab was struck in the rear by a light truck. The accident occurred on the Public Square, within view of my office window, while I was observing traffic. The truck backed to the curb and parked. The taxicab drifted backward and was stopped when a pedestrian opened the door and put on the brake. The woman was lifted from the cab in a limp condition and was placed on the sidewalk. An ambulance took her to Mercy Hospital. After the taxi drifted backward, I observed the exact outline of her car on the pavement at the site of collision by the dry dirt that had been knocked from underneath it by the force of the impact. I was on service at the hospital at the time and later was notified of her admission.

Examination disclosed a whiplash injury to the neck, with sprained ligaments and concussion of the cervical portion of the spinal cord. Roentgenograms revealed no abnormality. She was hospitalized for four weeks.

Sacroiliac pain on the right side developed one week later with referred pain into the outer side of the right thigh and leg as she became more active. A diagnosis of shearing injury to the right posterior sacroiliac ligament was made. She was given eight injections in five weeks, resumed her former activities in three months and remained cured for eight years.

In June 1952 the symptoms recurred when she bent forward to lift something from the bottom of a barrel. She stated that she had felt a "snap" in her right hip and severe pain similiar to that which she had had before. Two injections into the right posterior sacroiliac ligament failed to give the customary relief. After the third injection, upward traction on the extremity with the knee and hip flexed and the patient in the supine position apparently reduced what appeared to be a slight subluxation and assisted in the cure. At the time of writing, she has been entirely free from pain and has been performing her usual activities for five years. She was last seen in December 1956.

Case 4. In February 1951, a housewife, aged 56, was a passenger in the front seat of an automobile involved in a head-on collision. Her injuries were concussion of the brain and a contusion of the head, the impact shattering the windshield. She was hospitalized for two days and in bed for one week at home, and she was inactive for several weeks.

As activity increased, pain developed in the left sacroiliac joint. The first examination, in December 1951, revealed relaxation of the left posterior sacroiliac ligament of 10 months' duration, which had not been diagnosed. Referred pain extended into the posterolateral surface of the thigh and the outer side of the leg to within two inches of the external malleolus.

The pain was relieved by injection of a local anesthetic. Complete relief was obtained after six injections of a proliferating solution, and one month later the patient made a 5,000 mile automobile trip without discomfort. At the time of writing she has remained free from trouble for four years. She was last seen in October 1955.

Case 5. On June 9, 1953, a housewife, aged 58, missed the second step of a ladder and fell to the floor in a sitting position. She was confined to bed at home for two weeks under the care of the family physician with pain referred into the buttock, posterior thigh and the calf of the left leg. She was unable to take a step away from the bed or to bear any weight on the left foot. She was taken to the hospital by ambulance. On the day of admission, local anesthetic infiltration of the left posterior sacro-iliac ligament gave relief, and she took a few steps. Roentgenograms of the pelvis by the Chamberlain technic as described by Anderson and Peterson revealed the left pubes to be higher than the right. There was no fracture.

Six injections of proliferating solution were given in an eight-day period, and the patient returned home by automobile on the ninth day. Six days later she walked into my office, and a few days later drove 100 miles, returning home two days later.

Three weeks after leaving the hospital she was given one injection of proliferating solution and two weeks later drove 3,000 miles to California, returning by automobile after one month.

At the time of this report she is doing all her housework and has remained free from discomfort for three and one-half years. The last contact was in November 1956.

Case 6. A painter, aged 37, had a fall in which he fractured his skull and sprained his ankle. Three months later sacroiliac disability was diagnosed. He received eight injections in five weeks. He has remained cured for 16 years. His last examination was in December 1956.

Case 7. A railroad engineer, aged 63, was thrown from his engine and fractured his sacrum. Six months later bilateral sacroiliac disability was diagnosed. During a seven-week period, he received six injections on the left side and eight injections on the right. He has remained cured for 14 years. He was last seen in November 1954.

Case 8. A housewife, aged 49. No history of trauma. Her symptoms had lasted for 11 years. She had undergone hysterectomy and bilateral salpingectomy one year before examination, but these procedures had not affected her low-back pain. She had eight injections during a period of five weeks into her sacroiliac ligaments bilaterally and has remained cured for nine years. Her last examination was in May 1954.

Case 9. A farmer, aged 44. His symptoms, of two years duration, had begun while he was carrying a hog downstairs. He was unable to do light work. After seven sacroiliac intraligamentous injections within one month he was able to run a tractor with a plow attached and to reach all levers. He was last seen in September 1956, and he has been cured for 12 years.

Case 10. A tire-builder, aged 42. Gave a history of no injury but for 14 years had a gradually developing pain in his low back while handling tires in a stooped position. The pain was referred into both groin and the anterior upper thigh sometimes on one side or the other, or both. None in the extremities.

Examination revealed relaxation of the lumbosacral, iliolumbar and upper portion of the sacroiliac ligaments on both sides.

He received three injections in the lumbosacral ligaments, two in each iliolumbar, four in the right sacroiliac and three in the left sacroiliac ligaments over a period of 10 weeks. He has remained cured for six years. He was last seen in June 1955.

Case 11. An executive, aged 30. His symptoms, which had lasted for eight years, had begun while he was doing the high jump at college. Three years later they had been aggravated when he was loading a quarter of beef. He had five injections into the right sacroiliac ligaments within three weeks. He has remained cured for eight years. He was last seen in January 1955.

Case 12. Male clerk, aged 25. He developed a pain in the center of the low-back seven years previously, which was worse after bending or sitting. Eight months previous to examination, he received a severe jerk while lifting in a stooped position, and the pain had been more severe ever since. There was referred pain a short distance across his back at the lumbosacral level, but none in the buttock or legs.

Examination revealed trigger point pain in the lumbosacral depression, none on either side.

Three injections into the interspinus ligament were given over a period of four weeks while he continued his regular work. He has remained cured for nine years and resumed playing golf which he was unable to do before. Last examination was January 1957.

Case 13. A schoolboy, aged 15, the youngest patient in this series. His symptoms, of 15 months' duration, had resulted from an automobile accident. He received six injections in the left sacroiliac joint ligaments within three weeks and was cured. In another automobile accident two years later he sustained a fractured skull but no sacroiliac disability. He has remained cured for 11 years. His last examination was in June 1955.

Case 14. A retired insurance salesman, aged 81. He had developed a gradual weakness with increasing pain low in his back on the left side, over a period of 10 years, with no history of trauma. Stooping, lifting or walking gave a severe pain in the left buttock and referred into the outer side of the left leg.

Examination revealed a relaxation of the left posterior sacroiliac ligament. He was given six injections over a four-week period with complete relief. He is able to lift his invalid wife and sister without discomfort and has remained cured for three and one-half years. Last examination was in November 1956.

Case 15. A housewife, aged 29. During her first pregnancy five days before delivery, she developed a severe pain in the right sacroiliac area which was constant until delivery during any activity. She remained in bed three days without pain. On regaining her feet, the pain returned and had remained severe for eight months, causing a marked list of the body to the opposite side. There was referred pain to the outer side of the right leg. She consulted an orthopedic specialist on two occasions without benefit. The possibility of a disc operation and spinal fusion was discussed.

Five injections into the right sacroiliac ligaments entirely eliminated the pain and body list. Three weeks later she made a 1,500 mile automobile trip and played golf. She has had two children since. She has been entirely well for ten years. Her last examination was in December 1956.

Case 16. A housewife, aged 39, no children. She had severe low-back pain on both sides for nine years following a fall from a chair. Had been twice in a university hospital, and a complete hysterectomy had been performed. There was no relief.

She entered the hospital in an ambulance. Examination revealed a bilateral sacroiliac weakness. Nine injections were given in the sacroiliac ligaments during an eight-day stay in the hospital. She returned home in a car. Later she received four more injections in the office. Six injections were given in the left sacroiliac ligaments and seven in the right during a period of 15 days. She remained free from pain for three years.

During a course of six shock treatments in another city, she received a compression fracture of the body of the 3rd dorsal vertebra and was treated by hyperextension with good union of the fracture. It showed only slight compression one year later, but she had a very annoying pain in the region of the fracture during any activity and after sitting. There was referred pain laterally a few inches which was worse on the left side extending to the medial border of the scapula.

Examination revealed a relaxation of the supra and interspinus ligaments beneath the 2nd and 3rd dorsal spines. Three injections at two week intervals completely eliminated the pain, and she has been free from discomfort for three years. She was last seen in May 1955.

Case 17. Laborer, aged 48. Low back pain for 16 years and worse for two years following automobile accident. Had disc operation one year ago by neuro-ortho team. Report of three discs removed.

Pain always more severe on right side of pelvis than left or center, and referred pain never extended below the calf of either leg. Never had any pain in the lumbar area. Unable to work since operation, and steel brace did not benefit much. Leg pains unchanged following operation, but had additional severe constant pain entirely across the lumbar back and over the sacrum. Trigger point tenderness over both sacroiliac joint ligaments was confirmed by needling as was also the transverse processes of the 2-3-4-5 lumbar vertebrae on the left side and the 3-4-5 on the right side, and over the 1-2-3 sacral segments.

NOTE: Apparently the sacrospinalis muscle tendons were torn loose from the transverse processes of the lumbar vertebrae and sacrum while obtaining exposure during the operation. This frequently happens in the search for obscure suspected discs. In addition, there is often an extension or increase of sciatic pain into the feet from "freeing" radicular nerves of bony "impingement," or "adhesions" at subsequent search and fusion operations.

Prolotherapy partially relieved both lumbar sacral and extremity pains as revealed at a two-month check-up. Additional treatment should result in further improvement, but complete satisfactory recovery is not to be expected. The patients, however, are grateful for any noticeable improvement.

Case 18. A restaurateur, age 42. Low back pain 14 years on left side only, extending only to left calf. Operation 7 years ago at internationally-known clinic by neurological surgeon. Reported three discs removed. No improvement. Wears back support.

Since the operation he has the same pain in the left buttock extending into the left calf that was present before the operation. He has a new pain on the right side which extends back of the right knee gripping the calf of the right leg and extending beneath the arch of the right foot. It also is present on the top of the foot and extends into the 2-3-4 toes. There is also an additional pain in the left lumbar area extending to the lateral side of the back. Needling reproduced the pain in the left transverse processes of lumbar vertebra 2-3-4-5, and interspinus ligaments lumbar 2-3-4, but there was no trigger point tenderness nor needle tenderness of lumbar 5 interspinus space. Sacroiliac tenderness and needling pain were present on the lift side but not on the right.

Note: Apparently during the operation, the sacrospinus tendons had been torn from the transverse processes of the lumbar vertebra on the left side, the ligaments with their nerves had been extirpated from the 5th lumbar space, and the normal lumbar radicular nerves on the right side had been disturbed into a pathological condition to account for the sciatic pain in his right leg and foot, for which there is probably no relief.

The patient has been treated for the relaxed tendons from the lumbar transverse processes and for the relaxed left sacroiliac and iliolumbar ligaments, and he is now under observation.

Case 19. A housewife, aged 32, and mother of three children nine, six and four years of age. She gave a history of pain for two years in the coccyx when sitting. It was very severe for six months and was aggravated by riding in an automobile. For the first visit to the office, she reclined in the back seat of the car for the eight-mile drive.

She was given three treatments at seven-day intervals because she wanted to go on a family vacation automobile trip. One week after the third treatment she was free from pain and started on a 1,200 mile automobile trip which was completed in three weeks, free from pain. She has remained cured for four years, and her last examination was in September 1956. (Note: I have not removed a coccyx for 19 years.)

Case 20. A mailman, aged 30. Six years service on route with 1,335 steps to climb. Former basketball player and four and one half years in the U. S. Army. No history of any accident. On April 6, 1953, he first reported pain of three months duration in the left hip with increasing severity on walking up steps. He was free from pain on sitting except when leaning forward sorting mail.

Examination revealed trigger point tenderness over the hip joint posteriorly. There was pain on rotation of the hip joint when reclining with hip and knee flexed. When he climbed a step in the office, I could palpate a slight "slip" of the head of the femur as he raised his weight on the left foot. He was unable to work.

Four injections of the proliferating solution at weekly intervals were made within the articular ligament of the hip joint at the posterior superior margin. He returned to light work one month after completion of treatment, and two weeks later to the same route with 1,335 steps.

In December 1955 he slipped on the ice while carrying a load of mail and received a severe injury to the ligaments that support the left sacroiliac joint. It remained so painful and disabling that I treated the left posterior sacroiliac, sacrospinus and sacrotuberus ligaments one month later, and he returned to work in another month. There was no injury to the left hip ligaments. Examination in March 1957 revealed complete recovery, and he is working steadily carrying mail. The hip has now remained cured for four years.

Case 21. A nurse-secretary, aged 25. She had an injury to the left wrist three years previously with frequent recurring periods of severe pain which was most severe on full flexion of the wrist. It prevented typing, opening desk drawers, etc. A metal re-inforced leather brace gave relief and permitted working. Recurrences continued on removing the brace.

Examination revealed tenderness on light pressure over the dorsal surface of the left trapezoid bone as the wrist approached full flexion, which forced the trapezoid bone against the disabled dorsal ligament of the wrist and put the ligament under tension.

Three injections of the proliferant were made at the fibro-osseous attachment of the ligament as it passed over the bone. The patient has enjoyed full use of the wrist for four years without any return of pain. The last examination was in October 1957.

Case 22. A steel worker, aged 38. He suffered an injury to the external lateral ligament of the right ankle seven months previously when he stepped into a hole. The pain would frequently be accentuated by "turning" the ankle. An elastic brace gave relief. Three injections of the proliferant into the anterior branch of the ligament and two into the inferior branch, at two week intervals, strengthened the "weld" at the fibro-osseous attachment. There has been no recurrence in four years. His last examination was in January 1957.

Case 23. A school teacher, single, aged 29. Three automobile injuries in which she had either been thrown out, turned over, or struck in the rear with such force that she was unconscious from a whiplash injury to the neck. There were no fractures in any of the accidents.

Examination revealed a general joint relaxation throughout her body (loose-double jointed). X-rays were negative for any pathology, but her relaxed painful ligaments with unstable joints and pain involved cervical 1-2-3-4-5, dorsal 1-2-4-5-6-7, lumbar 3-4-5, bilateral sacroiliac, sacrococcygeal, and the right hip. There were 14 interspinus and articular ligaments involved, 2 iliolumbar, 2 posterior sacroiliac, one sacrospinus and sacrotuberus, one sacrococcygeal, and one articular ligament of the hip.

Her referred pains extended into her head, arm, fingers, into the groin, vagina, thigh, calf beneath heel and instep, and into toes. Her neck snapped on movement, and she had been unable to work for nine months since the last accident.

During four hospitalizations in a period of six months, she received a total of 85 treatments, made a satisfactory recovery, and returned to regular school teaching three months after the last treatment and has continued for two years.

(Caution:—Loose-jointed individuals should not get rolled in convertibles nor hit in the rear.)

Case 24. Foreman, aged 64. Pain for one year following an accident in which he was thrown spraining his right thigh high up inside where it became black and blue and resulted in pain ever since, although he kept working. Pain most severe next to the pelvis inside the thigh. Pain referred into the lower inside thigh and inside the leg anteriorly below the knee. He has limped ever since the accident, and herpes were present inside the lower half of the thigh. The calf of the right leg was one-half inch smaller than the left.

Trigger point tenderness was present at the tendenous attachment of the adductor muscles to the descending ramus of the pubic bone. Needling confirmed the diagnosis of tendon relaxation. Prolotherapy was followed by disappearance of the herpes in two weeks. A second treatment was given six weeks later when his condition had greatly improved. He has remained free of pain for six months.

Case 25. Physician, aged 68. Low back pain all his life. Worse for nine years following a severe twist. Pain was in the center and worse on bending over and riding in automobile. Constipated all his life with gas discomfort in lower abdomen. Had headaches. Was treated in Boston for adrenal insufficiency.

Ligament injection of lumbar 4 and 5 articulations reproduced pain. Prolotherapy of lumbar 4 and 5 interspinus articular and iliolumbar ligaments not only relieved the low back pain but also the constipation, abdominal gas disturbance and headaches following one treatment one year ago. Without taking any laxative as before, his bowels move twice daily.

Case 26. Wife of physician (Case 25), aged 59, no children. Low back pain 31 years. Worse on bending and stooping. Sometimes she made her bed on her knees.

Lumbar 4 and 5 joint instability verified by intraligamentous needling along with sacroiliac bilateral instability. Treatment at same time as her husband improved the stability of her joints as well as curing her constipation and abdominal discomfort from gas.

Later she received additional ligament treatment on two occasions of lumbar 2-3-4-5, cervical 4-5-6, dorsal 3-4-11, sacrococcygeal, and left ankle, and she has remained cured for six and one-half months since last treatment.

NOTE: This was my first inclination that abnormal somatic sensory stimulation of the ligaments that support the lumbosacral articulation reflexly affected the normal activity of the large intestine. During the past year I have observed it so many times that there can be no doubt of its existence. I have also observed the relation between the interspinus and articular ligaments of dorsal 12 and lumbar 1 and the referred complication of gas-constipation.

Case 27. Boat pilot, aged 41. Pain in back of neck for four years more on the left side going up in the back of the head on the left side and into the left eye. Needling reproduced pain in cervical 2-3-4 area. X-rays were negative. Prolotherapy within the interspinus ligaments and articular cervical ligaments on the left side relieved the pain. Treatment six weeks later was followed by considerable relief. Patient is now under observation.

Case 28. Farmer, aged 40. Fell from a roof 18 years ago followed by constant pain in neck radiating into above the spine of the right scapula, skips the shoulder, extends down the anterior surface of the arm, elbow and forearm, skips the wrist and hand, and is more severe in the second than the first and third fingers.

Needling the 7th cervical interspinus and more particularly the articular ligament on the right side reproduced the pain. He had much improvement following the first treatment and will return for further observation following the second treatment.

NOTE: Severe cervical joint instability, particularly if there is radiating pain to the head and upper extremities, almost invariably involves the articular ligaments along with the interspinus ligament. Head pain (eyes and temples) frequently results from tendon relaxation at the occipital ridge.

Case 29. Housewife, aged 52. Fell two years previously and injured her right shoulder. She was unable to raise her arm or put her hand up her back. She was unable to lie on it comfortably, and when lying on her left side, there was a pain when the right arm pulled on the shoulder.

Examination revealed tenderness at the tendon attachment of the deltoid muscle to the margin of the acromium process. Needling confirmed the diagnosis of relaxation of the tendon.

The pain was relieved after the second treatment, and after a few weeks full function was restored. There has been no recurrence in two years.

Case 30. Housewife, aged 36. Her left shoulder was injured one year previously when a large rolling door fell over against the back of the shoulder at an airport. It had become swollen and discolored, followed by pain on movements of the arm and scapula with limited function. Trigger points of pain were located over the supraspinatus and infraspinatus muscles.

Needling confirmed the diagnosis of tendon relaxation of the muscles at their attachments to the scapula.

Two treatments of the proliferant distributed against the bone beneath the muscles at a monthly interval entirely cleared up the condition, and she has resumed all usual activities for eighteen months without recurrence.

Case 31. Widow, aged 82, one child. Had "sciatica" nine years previously. Four months previous to examination she got a pain on top of the foot and into the toes. Needling verified pain in the right sacroiliac and right hip ligaments. There was sciatic nerve tenderness and a body list. She hobbled with a cane. The right ankle jerk was absent.

After two treatments of the sacroiliac ligaments and two of the hip, she made a full recovery, went on picnics, and felt like dancing after three months. No recurrence in two years.

Case 32. Electrician, aged 48. Low back pain 17 years, left more than right. For years he had rolled out of bed on knees and helped himself up with his arms on the bed. Slept for years on a bed board. For three months he slept on the floor. He would rather stand than sit and have to get up.

After one treatment to the sacroiliac ligaments on both sides, he was much better, and a relaxed gluteal tendon was located on the right side which was treated along with the sacrospinus and sacrotuberus ligaments on both sides. On the third visit he was still better, and a relaxed gluteal tendon on the left side was treated along with the left sacroiliac ligaments. Later the right gluteal tendon was treated. He made a complete recovery over a three-month period and has remained well for three years.

Case 33. Attorney, (golf-crazed) aged 53. Constant back pain for 37 years. Severe in summer from golfing. Spinal fusion operation in 1925 in New York extending from dorsal 9 to lumbar 1. Second spinal fusion operation extending from lumbar 5 to sacral 2 in 1951.

He first consulted me one year ago, and his relaxed ligaments were: interspinus and articular dorsal 1-4-5-6-11-12; lumbar 1-3-4-5; dorsal 8-9 rib tendons at internal rib angle and from body of 3rd right rib; iliolumbar ligaments right and left; sacroiliac ligaments right and left; sacrospinus and sacrotuberus ligaments right and left; tendons and fascia from posterior surface of greater trochanter of the right femur, and the adductor longus tendon from the right pubic bone.

After four treatments in four months he was much improved and put off treatments to play golf for five months. Two months ago I gave him 19 treatments on two consecutive days, and he will soon return for re-evaluation. (This case is mentioned to show the long period involving operations, the variety of fibrous tissue-skeletal disabilities that can befall one individual, and the retrogression of his condition by delaying treatment to participate inadvisedly in exercises.)

Case 34. A housewife and author, aged 37, and mother of three children, twelve, eight and three years of age. Her disability was of four years' duration with onset apparently caused by a severe cough. She had pain in the dorsal spine of the supraspinus and interspinus and left articular ligaments at D-4 and D-6 which radiated on the left side from D-6 to the medial border of the scapula. The pain was aggravated particularly when typing and washing dishes and was present everyday.

She received three injections at each dorsal interspace at three-week intervals. There was improvement of which she was aware following each treatment, and she has been free from symptoms for two years.

Case 35. European executive, aged 49. Severe low back pain eleven years, center and left side more than the right. Pain in both groin, and after driving had pain in back of right thigh. Worst was on bending. On awakening he had no idea whether he would be able to get out of bed, wash his face or get to the office without agony. He was unable to bend over billiard table, work in garden, or have intercourse. X-rays were negative.

Examination revealed relaxed ligaments of the 4th and 5th lumbar and bilateral sacroiliac joints. He was hospitalized, and on two successive days he was given a total of 20 injections within the ligaments. Because of the expense of making a second special trip for treatment, the Sylnasol solution was made up with equal parts of saline. His reaction was rather severe and remained in the hospital a total of two weeks after which he went shopping. He returned to Europe by plane after a few days in New York. A letter three weeks after the treatment reported he was going to work.

Within another month his back was stronger, and he was living a normal life including his sex activity. Within another month he was briskly swinging two suitcases in a London Railway station according to a relative. Later on he won the club billiard tournament.

Eight months after his treatment, he met me in Lisbon. He reported that he felt better than he had for eleven years and was not wearing a belt or brace. Examination revealed some tenderness of lumbar 3-4-5 and the upper sacroiliac ligaments. Because of business commitments, he decided to delay the treatment and have it given by my conferee in Lisbon, who is successfully carrying out the procedure. I report this case to show that stronger solutions of the proliferant may be used when circumstances warrant it.

Case 36. Retired executive, aged 77. Low back pain 56 years from catching his fiancée as she sprang from a buggy, and he attempted with one foot on the terrace to swing her over the mud to a walk. His foot slipped and he has had a constant disability with exacerbations ever since. His worst trouble was stooping over to pack a bag on his annual world cruises or lifting a bag. There is no other work that he is required to do.

I met him in the Canary Islands two years ago. Examination revealed a relaxation of the right sacroiliac ligaments. I applied his belt low over the pubes, and it gave relief while packing his bags. He visited me eight months later and I gave him five injections in the right sacroiliac ligaments. During the injection the point of the needle slipped into the sacroiliac joint three times. I withdrew it and changed to contact bone before injecting the proliferating solution. This indicates the considerable relaxation of the ligament and the instability of the joint. He has never had a headache in his life, and he has not had any referred pain from the sacroiliac disability.

He drove eighty miles that day and started driving to Arizona with his wife the next day.

Six months later he returned. His condition had improved considerably. I repeated the five injections. He took one small dose of analgesic and started driving for Maine the next day.

One year later I have just received a letter from Hong Kong stating that he is fine, but will stop again for a treatment to make him perfect. He has never taken any pain pills except the one in my office.

I mention this case to show how long these cases may persist and how much relaxation may be present in a patient with a high threshold of pain without having any referred pain or being entirely disabled and still have a constant disability. The examiner can often be misled by depending on the amount of the patient's complaint. These cases require more treatment than one would ordinarily expect. The history of headaches is very important—both ways.

Case 37. Housewife, aged 36, three children ages 11 to 16. Pain in the neck for two years following a rear-end automobile collision. The neck pain was in the center and right side accompanied by headache and referred pain to the right forehead and in the right eye, pain into the right arm and forearm anterolaterally and into the thumb, first and second fingers. All were aggravated by activity.

Examination revealed trigger point tenderness of the occipital bone on the right side which, on deep pressure, reproduced pain in the right eye. There was tenderness of the cervical 3rd, 4th, 5th and 6th vertebrae in the center and on the right side; none in the left.

Needling of the occipital bone one inch right of center reproduced pain in the right eye. Needling of the right articular ligaments on the lamina and transverse processes of the cervical 4th, 5th and 6th vertebrae reproduced the pain in the right thumb, first and second fingers.

Following prolotherapy of the occipital tendons and cervical ligaments, the referred pain into the right eye and right digits never recurred.

Following the second treatment two months later, the occipital, neck, arm pain, and headaches entirely cleared up. Has resumed normal activities and has been free from pain for one year.

Case 38. Loose-jointed housewife, aged 34, who grew up in a sheltered life. Two children ages 8 and 11 years. Never had a back pain until nine months previous to examination following her first golf lesson. Played golf throughout the summer. X-rays had been interpreted as "double-jointed lumbosacral articulation which should have given trouble all her life." Fitted with steel brace by two orthopedic surgeons and advised "to return for operation if not improved."

Low back pain worse in left lumbar area than right and concentrated above left anterior superior spine. No referred pain into the extremities.

To avoid unbearable pain she had slept for the previous three months on her left side on a narrow couch so that she could not turn over in her sleep.

Examination revealed relaxed tendons of left ribs 11 and 12; transverse processes of left dorsal 12; left and right lumbar 1, 2, 3, 4, and 5; left gluteal. The relaxed ligaments were 5th lumbar supra- and interspinus; left and right iliolumbar; left posterior sacroiliac; sacrospinus and sacrotuberus; right posterior sacroiliac (high only).

She received three series of treatment in the office at two month intervals while staying in a hotel across the street. Fifteen injections were given on two succeeding days in the first series, twenty-three injections in two days in the second series, and fourteen injections in two days in the third series. She has completely recovered, does her own housework, sleeps with her husband, and enjoys living. She has no desire to resume golf.

More treatments were necessary in the second series because re-examination after marked improvement revealed additional relaxed tendons and ligaments which were previously masked by the severe tenderness of the others.

This case is reported to reveal what can happen later in life to a loose-jointed individual who "grows up" without participating in tendon and ligament strengthen developing exercises. The loose-jointed type should engage daily in planned activities from the age of 5 to 22 years.

In such cases, a spinal fusion operation is contraindicated, devastating, unsuccessful, and is to be condemned.

Case 39. Factory bench worker and motorcycle racer, aged 24. Bilateral shoulder dislocation in motorcycle accident 5½ years ago. Each redislocated approximately 30 times. Reduces them himself. Assisted from bed by mother if it occurs in his sleep. Unable to throw a ball or sleep with hand under pillow. Most frequently occurs when stooped over and reaching under workbench to retrieve an object from the floor.

Trigger point pain and tenderness bilaterally for 5½ years beneath acromium process posteriorly and at anatomical neck of humerus posteriorly where the supra- and infraspinatus tendons are attached as they reinforce the capsular ligament.

Prolotherapy to both trigger points bilaterally.

Six weeks later the trigger point pain and tenderness had disappeared, obviating the advisability of a second treatment. Went through all previously restricted movements without discomfort. Lost one week from work. Is riding his motorcycle. Will enter races in a few months.

MATERIAL USED BY THE AUTHOR

Proliferating Solutions

    (1) Sylnasol, 60 cc. vial.

        (G. D. Searle & Co., P.O. Box 5110, Chicago 80, Ill.)

    (2) Zinc sulfate-phenol Stock solution.

Zinc sulfate	8 Grams
Liquid Phenol	12 cc.
Glycerin	24 cc.
Dist. Water add to	100 cc.

        Mix solution for injection as follows:

Zinc sulfate-phenol stock	4 cc.
Pontocaine, 0.15%	42 cc.
Normal Saline	42 cc.

Anesthetic Solution

    Pontocaine, 0.15%, 100 cc. vial.

    (Winthrop Lab., 1450 Broadway, New York City)

Syringes

    Luerlock, 2 cc., 5 cc., 10 cc.

Needles

    Luerlock, Safety (bead on Barrel): 22 gauge—1 inch, 1½ inch, 2 inch, 2½ inch, 3 inch.

    (Becton, Dickinson & Co., Rutherford, New Jersey.)

Electric Needle Sharpener

    Such as "Guild" Pointer.

Skeleton

    Spine and pelvis—plastic.

    (Clay-Adams Co., 141 East 25th St., New York City.)

Anatomy Textbook

Sacroiliac Belt

(For all sacroiliac cases following treatment.)
1. Hackett Sacroiliac Belt.
   (S. H. Camp & Co., Jackson, Michigan)
2. Man's trouser belt, such as regular web U. S. Army belt.

Shoulder Brace

Model 53 (for upper dorsal ligament and tendon strain.)
(S. H. Camp & Co., Jackson, Michigan.)

Crutches

Following treatment for all cases with sciatica.
(A cane does not sufficiently relieve strain on ligaments.)

Written Post-treatment Instructions

(Sample below.)

INSTRUCTIONS FOR PATIENTS AFTER RECEIVING TREATMENT TO STRENGTHEN THEIR BACK LIGAMENTS AND TENDONS

* A reaction is necessary to cure this disability.

* Take pain pills with a full glass of water when you first become uncomfortable. Repeat in one hour if pain is not relieved. Continue taking it often enough to control pain as many days as it lasts. (It is easier to stop pain before it becomes severe.)

* If nauseated or dizzy, remain in bed. Use towel rather than get up to bathroom. Sip boiling (thermos bottle) water for hours. After hot water, try ginger ale. Avoid fruit or fruit juices. Dramamine, 50 mg., may be given every 4 to 6 hours for vomiting.

* Hot beverages assist absorption of medicine, empties stomach and allays nausea. Drink enough liquids to keep urine clear.

* Rub area well with liniment three times a day, then apply heating pad. It relieves pain and prevents muscle spasm. You will begin to get relief sometimes after the second day. Everybody's reaction varies. Continue the medication until you are comfortable. You may be aware of benefit before one month, but do not attempt to come to any conclusion regarding your condition until after two months.

* Diet: For a few days, no fruit juices. Eat very lightly, preferably hot foods.

* On third day it is advisable to take a saline cathartic, such as Sal Hepatica. Get daily elimination.

Return to light work when able. But for six weeks avoid such activities as bending, lifting, sweeping, ironing, raking, mowing, shoveling, bowling, golf, or any of your usual work that brought on pain before or now.

Exercises further weaken relaxed ligaments. After treatment, exercises interfere with new tissue becoming strong throughout the six weeks while it is forming.

If you have a brace or belt, you may wear it for 6 weeks, particularly while working. A man's belt pulled tight below the abdomen at the pubic bone level frequently is better than any other belt for weak sacroiliac ligaments, but the wider brace with supports is better for weak lumbar (small of the back) ligaments.

Your disability of weak ligaments, which stretched under strain, permitted traction on the sensory nerves, giving rise to pain.

We performed experiments on rabbits. They revealed the strength of the ligaments was doubled by action of the medicine.

Many patients are anxious to know how the treatment works. The medicine is injected into the ligament. It remains there several weeks, and by irritation it stimulates the formation of new bone and fibrous tissue which strengthens the ligament permanently (similar to the formation of a pearl in an oyster.)

We are anxious for you to make a complete recovery and be able to do anything you ever did before without having any pain or recurrence. 82% of our patients have made complete recoveries without recurrence for periods up to 18 years. (Every golfer hits the ball farther after his pelvis is stabilized). Over 1500 patients have been treated without any unfavorable result.

Come back at each appointment for a check-up. The examination will disclose whether further treatment is necessary. Continue with us until you are cured. Then report to us by visit or letter. We are interested in you.

Any physician can learn the diagnosis and treatment from the book, "Ligament and Tendon Relaxation Treated by Prolotherapy", (3rd Edition) G. S. Hackett, M.D., F.A.C.S., published by Charles C Thomas Co., Springfield, Illinois.. It is the only book ever written about ligaments. After you are benefitted, contact every physician you know and tell them about the book and the treatment, so they can benefit others. Tell them they are welcome to visit our office to learn the technic.

BACK EXERCISES

(To be started 6 weeks after back injection)

For six weeks following treatment you are to avoid any unnecessary exercises or activities. This includes any part of your regular work that brings on pain. It takes six weeks for the new tissue to become strong.

Beginning six weeks after treatment, gradual daily exercises will overcome much of the tired, stiff and aching feeling in your body and extremities.

Just as an athlete gradually gets into condition, the exercises will build up the previously weakened muscles, ligaments, tendons and joints after they have been sufficiently strengthened by the treatment.

All movements in the following exercises are to be done *slowly*. *Relax* between each movement, and never go far enough to produce pain.

1. Lie on your stomach with your arms to your sides. Raise the head and shoulders until you feel a slight pull in the low back. Hold this position 15 or 20 seconds, then let down. Repeat 2 or 3 times. Also while on your stomach, keep your legs straight and raise one at a time alternately.

2. Stand with your knees straight and feet together. Bend forward until you feel some pull in the small of your back. Straighten up and bend backward to where it becomes uncomfortable. Come back to a standing position.

3. Stand with your hands behind your head. Push backward with your head against your hands until you feel a pull down your back.

4. Stand with hands behind the head, the elbows pulled backward. Rotate shoulders and elbows to the right and left, keeping hips and knee straight and stationary.

5. Stand erect. Bend to the side, right and left.

You should go through these procedures 2 or 3 times a day. Increase 1 each day until you are doing 12 to 15, twice a day. Later you may gradually increase, but *never to where pain is produced*. These exercises should be kept up for perhaps 6 months to a year. If you wish to keep your back strong, you should do them at least 10 or 12 times once a day as long as you feel the need for them.

If your back does not respond favorably after one month of exercises, you should return for an examination to determine your condition. Additional treatment might be advisable.

BIBLIOGRAPHY

ALPERS, B. J.: The Problem of Sciatica. *M. Clin. North America,* *37*:503-510, 1953.

ANDERSON, R., AND LAUGHLIN, I.: The Management of Backache. *M. Clin. North America, 37*:No. 4 (July) 1953.

ARMSTRONG, J. R.: The Causes of Unsatisfactory Results From the Operative Treatment of Lumbar Disc Lesions. *J. Bone & Joint Surg., 33B1*:31-35 (Feb.) 1951.

BADGLEY, C. E.: Indications for Disc Operations. *Mod. Med.,* pp. 174, (Jan. 15) 1953.

BAER, W. S.: Sacro-Iliac Strain. *Bull. Johns Hopkins Hosp., 28*:159-163, 1917.

BARR, J. S.: Protruded Discs and Painful Backs. *J. Bone & Joint Surg., 33B1*:3-4, (Feb.) 1951.

BISTROM, O.: Degenerative Changes in the Spine and Back Pain. *Ann. chir. et gynaec. Fenniae, 43*:29, 1954.

BONICA, J. J.: *The Management of Pain.* Philadelphia, Lea, 1953.

BRAIN, W. R.: *Diseases of the Nervous System.* London, Oxford Univ. Press, 1951.

CHANDLER, F. A.: Trisacral Fusion; An Operative Technique Facilitating Combined Ankylosis of the Lumbosacral Joints of the Spine and Both Sacroiliac Joints. *Surg., Gynec., & Obst., 48*:501, 1929.

COMPERE, E. L.: Review and Editorial Comment. *Yearbook of Orthopedic and Traumatic Surgery,* pp. 154-55, 1956-57.

FRANCIS, C. C.: *The Human Pelvis.* St. Louis, Mosby, 1952, pp. 43-46.

GAENSLEN, F. J.: Sacroiliac Arthrodesis: Indications, Author's Technic and End-Results. *J.A.M.A., 89*:2031, (Dec. 10) 1927.

GARDNER, E.: Blood and Nerve Supply of Joints. *Stanford M. Bull., 11*:203 (Nov.) 1953.

GHORMLEY, R. K.: Backache: Examination and Differential Diagnosis. *J.A.M.A., 125*:412-416, 1944.

GHORMLEY, R. K.: An Etiologic Study of Backache and Sciatic Pain. *Proc. Staff Meet., Mayo Clinic, 26*:457-463, 1951.

GRANT, J. C.: *Bioleau, A Method of Anatomy.* 3rd Ed. Baltimore, Williams & Wilkins, 1944.

HACKETT, G. S.: Joint Stabilization Through Induced Ligaments Sclerosis. *Ohio State M. J., 49:*877 (Oct.) 1953.

HACKETT, G. S.: Shearing Injury to the Sacroiliac Joint. *J. Internat. Coll. Surgeons, 22:*631 (Dec.) 1954.

HACKETT, G. S.: Referred Pain From Low Back Ligament Disability. *A.M.A. Archives of Surg., 73:*878 (Nov.) 1956.

HACKETT, G. S.: Low Back Pain. *Brit. J. Phys. Med., 19:*25 (Feb.) 1956.

HACKETT, G. S.: Referred Pain and Sciatica in Low Back Diagnosis. *J.A.M.A., 163:*183, 1957.

HACKETT, G. S.: Ligament Relaxation and Osteo-Arthritis (Loose Jointed vs Close Jointed). *Rheumatism* (British), 1958.

HACKETT, G. S., AND HENDERSON, D. G.: Joint Stabilization. An Experimental, Histologic Study with Comments on the Clinical Application in Ligament Proliferation. *Am. J. Surg., 89:*968-973 (May) 1955.

HALL AND FRASER: Quoted by Riddle, P.: *Injection Treatment.* Philadelphia, Saunders Co., 1940, p. 3.

HARRIS, F. I., AND WHITE, A. S.: Injection Treatment of Hernia; Its Experimental Basis. *California & Western Med., 45:*382-385, 1936.

HARRIS, F. I., WHITE, A. S., AND BISKIND, G. R.: Observations on Solutions Used for the Injection Treatment of Hernia. *Am. J. Surg., 39:*112-119, 1938.

HEAD, SIR HENRY: On Disturbances of Sensation with Special Reference to Pain of Visceral Disease. *Brain, 16:*1, 1892.

JAYNES: Quoted by Riddle, P.: *Injection Treatment.* Philadelphia, Saunders, 1940.

JUDOVICH, B., AND BATES, W.: *Pain Syndromes.* 3rd Ed. Philadelphia, Davis, 1950.

LENNANDER, K. G.: Über die Sensebilitat der Bauchhohle und über lokale und allgemeine Anasthesie bei Bruchund Bauchoperationeu. *Zbl. Chir., 28:*209-223, 1901.

LERICHE, R.: Effets de l'anesthesia a la novocaine des ligaments et des insertion tendineuses periarticulaires dans certanes maladies articulaires et dans les vices de positions fonctionnels des articulations. *Gaz. d. Hop., 103:*1294, 1930.

LEWIN, P.: *Backache and Sciatic Neuritis.* Philadelphia, Lea, 1943.

LOWMAN, E. W.: Osteoarthritis. *J.A.M.A., 157:*487-488 (Feb. 5) 1955.

MACKENZIE, J.: Quoted by Bonica, J. J.: *The Management of Pain.* Philadelphia, Lea, 1953.

Magnuson, P. B.:   Differential Diagnosis of Causes of Pain in the Lower Back Accompanied by Sciatic Pain.   *Ann. Surg., 119*:878-891, 1944.

Maniol, L.:   Histologic Effects of Various Sclerosing Solutions Used in the Injection Treatment of Hernia.   *Arch. Surg., 36*:171-189, 1938.

Mayer, I.: Quoted by Riddle, P.: *Injection Treatment.*   Philadelphia, Saunders, 1940.

Meisenbach, R. O.:   Sacro-Iliac Relaxation With Analysis of Eighty-four Cases.   *Surg., Gynec., & Obst., 12*:411-434, 1911.

Mengert, W. F.:   Referred Pelvic Pain.   *Southern M. J., 36*:256-263, 1943.

Millikan, C. H.:   The Problem of Evaluating Treatment of Protruded Lumbar Intervertebral Disc.   *J.A.M.A., 155*:1141-1143, 1954.

Mixter, W. J., and Barr, J. S.:   Ruptured Intervertebral Disc with Involvement of Spinal Canal.   *New England J. Med., 211*:210-215 (Aug. 2) 1934.

Newman, P. H.:   Sacro-Iliac Arthrodesis.   *Proc. Roy. Soc. Med., 39*:715-718, 1945-1946.

Ober, F. R.:   The Role of the Iliotibial Band and Fascia Lata as a Factor in the Causation of Low Back Disabilities and Sciatica.   *J. Bone & Joint Surg., 18*:105, 1936.

Ober, Frank R.:   Lame Backs.   *Maine M. J., 44*:281 (Oct.) 1953.

O'Connell, J. E. A.:   Protusions of the Lumbar Intervertebra Discs.   *J. Bone & Joint Surg., 33B1*:8-30 (Feb.) 1951.

Rice, C. O.:   The Rationale of the Injection Treatment of Hernia.   *Minnesota Med., 18*:623-626, 1935.

Riddle, P.: *Injection Treatment.*   Philadephia, Saunders, 1940.

Ross, J.: Quoted by Bonica, J. J.: *The Management of Pain.*   Philadelphia, Lea, 1953.

Schultz, Louis W.:   A Treatment for Subluxation of the Temporomandibular Joint.   *J.A.M.A., 109*:1032, 1937.

Scuderi, C.:   Diagnosis and Treatment of Backache From the Standpoint of the General Practitioner.   *J. Oklahoma State M. A.*, pp. 191-197 (July) 1954.

Shands: *Handbook of Orthopedic Surgeon.*   4th Ed. St. Louis, Mosby, 1952.

Splithoff, C. A.:   Lumbo-Sacral Junction Roentgenographic Comparison of Patients With and Without Backache.   *J.A.M.A., 152*:1610 (Aug. 22) 1953.

STEINBROCKER, O.: Analgesic Block in the Diagnosis and Treatment of Low-Back Pain. Curr. Researches in *Anesth. & Analg., 20*:221-224, 1941.

STEINDLER, ARTHUR: Low Back Pain; An Anatomic and Clinical Study. *J. Iowa M. Soc., 15*:473 (Sept.) 1925.

STEINDLER, ARTHUR (In Collaboration with LUCK, J. V.): Differential Diagnosis of Pain Low in the Back; Allocation of the Source of Pain by the Procaine Hydrochloride Method. *J.A.M.A., 110*:106-113, 1938.

TRAVELL, J., AND TRAVELL, W.: Therapy of Low Back Manipulation and of Referred Pain in the Lower Extremity by Procaine Infiltration. *Arch. Phys. Med., 27*:537-547, 1946.

VELPEAU: Referred to by RIDDLE, P.: *Injection Treatment.* Philadelphia, Saunders, 1940.

WARREN, J. H.: *Hernia With Cure by Subcutaneous Injection.* Boston, Charles N. Thomas, 1881.

WATERS, C. H., JR.: Management of Acute Low Back Problems. *Nebraska State Med. J., 37*:205-240 (July) 1952.

INDEX